PHYSICIAN
OF THE SOUL

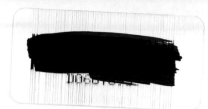

PHYSICIAN OF THE SOUL

A MODERN KABBALIST'S APPROACH TO HEALTH AND HEALING

by Rabbi Joseph H. Gelberman, Ph.D.
with Lesley Sussman

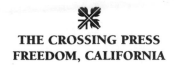

THE CROSSING PRESS
FREEDOM, CALIFORNIA

For information on bulk purchases or group discounts for this and other Crossing Press titles, please contact our Special Sales Manager at 800/777-1048.

Visit our Web site: www.crossingpress.com

Library of Congress Cataloging-in-Publication Data

Gelberman, Joseph H.
    Physician of the soul : a modern kabbalistic aproach to health and healing / by Joseph H. Gelberman.
        p. cm.
    ISBN 1-58091-061-0 (pbk.)
    1. Cabala--Health aspects. 2. Health--Religious aspects--Judaism 3. Mysticism--Health aspects. I. Title.

    RZ999.G35   2000
    615.8'52--dc21   99-058581

Dedicated to my father, Reb Dovid, who taught me all about growth and how to be alive and awake. And to all my great teachers in the yeshivas of Europe.

I want to thank Les Sussman, who patiently spent many hours listening to my stories and my teachings without any complaint or fidgeting. I also want to thank my beautiful wife, Jan, for all her patience and support during the writing of this book.

I sincerely want to thank all my students at the seminary and in my Kabbalah classes. They helped me to realize that each one of us is a Physician of the Soul. Let me also thank the Almighty, who, in the Bible, is described as "The Great Physician."

A great debt of gratitude is owed to my editor, Caryle Hirshberg, who understands the majesty of Kabbalah, and my agent, Claire Gerus, who is a spirit soul and a special friend.

Last, but not least, I want to thank all my friends everywhere in the world from Sri Swami Satchidananda to the good people at the Interfaith League of Devotees.

Special thanks to all of you affiliated with my synagogue in New York City who have been loyal and supportive all these years—especially my dear friend Rabbi Roger Ross, Rabbi Michael Shivack, and my devoted cantor, Judith Steel.

Table of Contents

Foreword by Sri Swami Satchidananda 13

Preface by Rabbi Gelberman 17

Author's Note 23

Introduction: What Is Kabbalah? 29

Chapter One: A Partnership with God 35

Chapter Two: The Tyranny of Fear 49

Chapter Three: Dethroning Fear 52

Chapter Four: Two Divinely Powerful Ladies 63

Chapter Five: Getting on the Right Road 71

Chapter Six: Purifying Body, Mind, and Soul 76

Chapter Seven: Moving Toward Wholeness 83

Chapter Eight: Healing Modalities. 92

Chapter Nine: The Way of the Mystic 102

Chapter Ten: The Tree of Life. 114

Chapter Eleven: The Healing Tree 126

Chapter Twelve: Three Case Histories 140

Chapter Thirteen: The Physician of the Soul. 147

Healing Prayers. 167

Glossary 171

Who Am I?

"I am the reality of things that seem
I am the waking who am called the dream
I am the utmost height there is to climb
I am stability, all else will pass
I am eternity circling time
Kill me, none may, conquer me, nothing can
I am God's soul fused in the heart of man."
                                    —Anonymous

Maimonides' Prayer for Healing

Exalted God, before I begin the holy work of healing the creations of your hands, I place my entreaty before the throne of your glory that you grant strength of spirit and fortitude to faithfully execute my work.

Let not desire for wealth or benefit blind me from seeing truth. Deem me worthy of seeing in the sufferer who seeks my advice a person—neither rich nor poor, friend or foe, good man or bad. Of a man in distress, show me only the man.

If doctors wiser than me seek to help me understand, grant me the desire to learn from them, for the knowledge of healing is boundless. But when fools deride me, give me fortitude!

Let my love for my profession strengthen my resolve to withstand the derision even of men of high station. Illuminate the way for me, for any lapse in my knowledge can bring illness and death upon your creations.

I beseech you, merciful and gracious God, strengthen me in body and soul, and instill within me a perfect spirit.

Foreword
by Sri Swami Satchidananda

I met Rabbi Gelberman in the mid-60s at a time when the youth of America was undergoing a radical change. This was at the height of the hippie movement and these young people were searching for the meaning of life and an understanding of the mysteries of the spirit. Rabbi was sharing the wisdom of the Kabbalah in New York and I was teaching Yoga there on the invitation of filmmaker Conrad Rooks and artist Peter Max.

We first met at a Yoga retreat in Val Morin, Canada. Rabbi Gelberman was offering a Sabbath service there and he invited me to attend and to say a few words after the service. I had never met a Rabbi before and was not sure what to expect. I was so delighted to see that we shared much in common. Later, in New York, as we exchanged ideas and spent time together, we were able to share the richness of our respective traditions. We developed a wonderful love and respect for one another. We decided to let that interfaith experience radiate outward and we invited other dear friends, Br. David Steindl-Rast and Shimano Roshi to join our discussion group that evolved into The Center for Spiritual Studies.

Together, over the years, we conducted interfaith programs, retreats, and worship services. During our services, we would sit together in a circle around a central light. Then, each of the clergy would offer worship according to his or her own tradition, to that central light. That light was a symbol of the Divine and we experienced what became my motto: "Truth is One, Paths are Many." We enjoyed this tremendously, and all those who witnessed these services experienced the joy that flowed from appreciating the unity within our diversities.

These services showed us that we each brought the unique language and symbols of our spiritual traditions to the common altar. And, like a bouquet of flowers has its various colors and fragrances, it was the magnificent variety that added to the beauty and charm of the arrangement. In this spirit of brother- and sisterhood and of interfaith cooperation, we developed a deep bond and lasting friendships.

Rabbi Gelberman and I continue to have a yearly program we call "The Swami and The Rabbi." These programs are a celebration of music and the philosophy of our traditions, which we both recognized, had deep reasonances and commonalties. At the heart of Judaism and the Kabbalah, as well as at the heart of Hinduism and Yoga, is the understanding that the mind, body, and spirit need to be in balance in order to experience that at-oneness, communion, union, nirvana, the Shekinah. And further, as Rabbi always points out, in his last life he was the Swami and I was the Rabbi! I always love that point!

I consider Rabbi Gelberman himself to be a physician of the soul. As a Rabbi, as a counselor, as a teacher and mentor, he has helped so many people find their way back to health, wholeness, and holiness. This wonderful book that Rabbi has written makes the ancient and mystical teachings of the Kabbalah very accessible to the reader.

Rabbi has lived and breathed Kabbalah so this is not a theoretical or philosophical text; rather he translates age-old precepts into profound insights that, when applied in one's daily life, can truly facilitate real health and healing. Rabbi Gelberman provides the readers with wonderful exercises and practical ways to apply these teachings. He teaches us how to "dethrone" fear, how to conduct a psychospiritual checkup, and how you can purify the mind and body and access the wisdom of the soul.

The teachings of the Kabbalah are a pathway to health and well-being. The difference between illness and wellness can be illustrated by the words themselves. Illness means that my vantage point of life is from a perspective of "I" or "I-Illness"; it bespeaks limitation and self-centeredness. When my approach to life is from a selfless perspective, there is "We" or "We-llness"; I am living an inclusive and interdependent life. I like to describe the goal of Yoga using three words: peaceful, easeful, useful. When you are in peace and at ease, you will be useful. And by living a dedicated, selfless life, you will enjoy supreme peace and joy.

This is the view of all the great world faiths and wisdom traditions; the purpose of religion is to help us lead a life that is loving, compassionate, and caring. In the Judeo-Christian tradition, we find the central precept, "Love thy neighbor as thyself." In Hinduism, we find the prayer, "Bandhava Siva Bhaktaha, Swadesho Bhuvana Tryam," which means: "All the peoples are my relatives, the entire universe is my home."

I see these same principles in the teachings of the Kabbalah and in the words of our beloved Rabbi. I am so happy that he has written such an enlightening book. Rabbi Gelberman encourages his readers in this wonderful book to affirm that: "We are ready to bring new life and health into being. We are more open, more accepting, more loving, more joyous, and more peaceful." May all the readers experience the health, healing, and joy that the mystical teachings of the Kabbalah and Physicians of the Soul have to offer them. Om Shanthi Shanthi Shanthi.

Sri Swami Satchidananda
Founder/Spiritual Head
Satchidananda Ashram and Integral Yoga Institutes
Headquarters: Yogaville, Virginia

Preface
by Rabbi Gelberman

I grew up in a nine-room brick house in Nageyched, Hungary, more than eighty years ago. It was a little village that had only dirt roads, so my shoes were always a little muddy. I was the ninth child of seventeen children, and my father was a rabbi who also ran the general store in this small town where Hassidism and Kabbalah both flourished.

Hassidism is a Jewish sect that has immersed itself in the study of mysticism dating back to eighteenth century Europe. The movement, with its emphasis on "inner truths," was founded by a great teacher and rabbi by the name of Israel Ben Eliezer. He is better known to the world as the Baal Shem Tov, meaning "the Master of the Good Name."

The study of Kabbalah runs deep in my family. My father, God bless his soul, was a Kabbalist, as was his father, and his father before him. I come from a line of Hassidim who were always involved in pursuing the mysteries of these ancient texts.

As a youngster and the son of a rabbi, I studied Kabbalah with masters of this mystical tradition at home and at the *yeshiva*, a Hebrew parochial school. This was in addition to my regular religious studies so that I could follow in my father's footsteps and become a rabbi.

I think that at age five I knew as many prayers as my elders. My primer was the *Torah*, the first five books of the Old Testament that were revealed by God to Moses.

However, it was my studies of the mysterious world of the Kabbalah with its *Etz Hayim*—the Tree of Life—as its primary symbol that most fascinated me.

At this early age I was already trying to fathom the meaning of the ten *sefiroth,* or spheres, located on the "branches" of this sacred tree. These studies were a mind-expanding introduction to Jewish mysticism. It is an inquiry to which I still dedicate my life.

In 1939, I found myself on the shores of America, a foreigner who spoke no English. I had left my wife, Yolan, and rosy-cheeked laughing baby, Judith, in Hungary to seek a job as a rabbi in this new land, praying that I would be successful in my job search and then earn enough money to bring my family to this country.

I was successful in my quest, finding a job at New York City's Congregation Zichron Efraim where I was paid $5 per week to be their rabbi. But by the time I had saved enough money to bring Yolan and Judith here, I no longer had a family. Letters suddenly stopped coming and after some frantic phone calls I was told that they had perished in a Nazi concentration camp at Auschwitz, Germany, "sometime in 1944."

America was good to me. I got my Bachelor's and Master's degrees at City College and continued my studies at Columbia University. I later went on to get my Doctorate in philosophy.

I eventually became a psychotherapist, studying under Dr. Nador Fodr, author of *The Search for the Beloved* and *A New Approach to Dream Interpretations.*

My interest in mysticism, however, never lagged, and my early background in Kabbalah led me to pursue other modern metaphysical approaches to religion.

I delved into the mysteries of Science of Mind, Unity, and Religious Science among other metaphysical systems. I also studied Eastern philosophies, such as yoga, and gained valuable and insightful experiences in various ashrams throughout the United States.

Today, I consider myself a "modern" Hassidic rabbi similar in beliefs and practices to Martin Buber. I am a modern rabbi living in a modern world who, in 1977, organized an interfaith temple and The New Seminary in New York City under the guidance of a swami, a priest, a minister, and a rabbi.

But despite such modernity, I also remain very much a part of Jewish tradition, whether that tradition has its roots in mysticism like the

Kabbalah, or more traditional outlets such as the Orthodox, Conservative, or Reformed movements of Judaism.

I will not turn my back on any of these approaches as long as they answer the following question: If I adhere to this, will it make me a better person, a better husband, a better neighbor, or a better rabbi?

I also apply the same high standard to other spiritual traditions I have studied over the years, including Christianity and Hinduism. All of these pursuits have been part of my lifelong quest to learn how to be "fully alive" on the physical, spiritual, and psychological levels; how to live in joy and harmony.

In this book I hope to share with you much of what I've learned from my study of Kabbalah, especially as it pertains to health and healing. If you are reading this book while suffering from some disease, I hope that what you learn here will give you the courage and confidence to become a physician of your soul and bring about a spiritual healing. If you are presently in good health, my fervent wish is that the lessons you learn here will help prevent the onset of any illness in the future.

One of the primary lessons of *Physician of the Soul* is that your body is not your enemy but a friend. If you fall ill, it may be that your body has somehow been neglected on some subtle physical, emotional, or spiritual energy level.

The importance of restoring harmony to these centers in order to maintain or regain health has been taught by healers of many spiritual traditions, for a long time.

Navajo Indian medicine men, for example, believe that the cure to illness lies in understanding the cause of illness and returning the body, mind, and soul to its natural equilibrium. This is a concept to which I subscribe as well.

Through a reading of this book you will begin the process of learning what may have gone wrong and ways to correct these deficient energy centers so that health-inducing harmony and balance can be restored to the body.

I must caution you, however, that while this book can be used as a powerful tool for healing, Kabbalah offers no miracle cure or quick fix approach to what ails you.

Nor is this book intended to replace your regular medical care. The

Kabbalistic techniques discussed here are to be used as an *addition*—not a substitute—for conventional medical treatment.

In this book you will gain a basic understanding of how the Tree of Life can be used to promote healing. You will also learn all about the invisible healing powers of the *Shekinah*, the feminine aspect of God that can be found within all of us, and the *Neshama*, the highest level of the multi-faceted soul.

You will learn about various spiritual illnesses, which can affect the body, soul, and mind, and discover ways to regain spiritual vitality. In addition, you will be taught various Kabbalistic meditations, visualizations, and affirmations. If used properly, they will offer powerful psychological and physical benefits.

Furthermore, you will gain a glimpse into the workings of the mind of the mystic, and discover how to utilize techniques such as the "mystical trance" to bring you closer to the true source of all healing—Almighty God.

One simple piece of advice, which is repeatedly found throughout this book, is the value of living life with joy and enthusiasm even in the face of adversity. Joy is centered inside where material possessions are not important.

Joy is not like happiness, which is outer-directed. It is only within ourselves that we can have a soul-to-soul encounter with the *Shekinah*, the indwelling spirit of God.

The study of Kabbalah is a lifelong commitment. It is a complex metaphysical system that includes the use of numbers—*gematria*—and the letters of the Hebrew alphabet, which are considered sacred by the Kabblistic mystics.

These fascinating aspects of Kabbalah are beyond the scope of this book. If, however, you are interested in delving deeper into such mysteries—and I highly recommend that you do—I would suggest books by Aryeh Kaplan, Dion Fortune, or Adolphe Franck.

Before we begin our healing journey through the world of the *Etz Hayim*, the Tree of Life, let me leave you with your first taste of Kabbalistic wisdom: The Bible said, "*Yom zeh orah v'simha, shalom umnacha.*"

In Hebrew, it means "this is a day of light and a day of joy, a day of peace and total harmony."

When the ancient mystics studied this phrase they asked: "What day was the Bible referring to?" The answer they received was, "This day! This is the only day we have. Yesterday is gone and tomorrow is uncertain."

No matter what the state of your health is, what is most important is that you do not worry about what happened yesterday or what might happen tomorrow. Yesterday is gone and tomorrow will take care of itself. Today is the day—the only day!

So, instead of worrying, affirm this day as the great gift from God that it is. When you do so, then the body is at rest and the mind is calmed so that it can receive spiritual wisdom. Your soul is better able to use her wings to fly higher to let God know that you are now ready to receive His/Her gift of healing.

Author's Note

The Tree of Life is a spiritual self-help manual that encourages us to utilize our intuition and imagination in seeking answers to the problems and challenges of everyday life.

There is no way around this process of "tuning in" if we are truly seeking a deeper awareness of who we are in the universe. The use of our intuitive faculties is also important for understanding the underlying causes of our illnesses.

These intuitive faculties help us bridge the gap between knowing something intellectually and experientially. For example, if you are ill your doctor can give you a pretty accurate diagnosis of what's wrong according to his or her medical books.

But unless you try to dig further you may be cured—your symptoms may go away—but you won't be healed. To be "healed" requires embarking on an intuitive quest that taps into the great mystical power of the Kabbalah.

It is through a study of Kabbalah and an understanding of the workings of the Tree of Life, that we can discover what subtle energy disorders and imbalances may have been responsible for the disease in the first place.

Without such knowing, the problem that led to your disorder will continue to fester. That is why the mystics believed that true healing had very little to do with fixing pain. They felt that only through soul work could imbalances be discovered and the real process of healing begin.

Many of you who are reading this book may already be familiar with some of the intuitive techniques we will be using in this book for our healing work—tools such as meditation, visualization, affirmations, and even prayer. If that is the case, you may skip the rest of this chapter and move on to the next.

For those readers who are new to such practices, I will briefly describe how each of these powerful transpersonal techniques works. By the way, none of these methods are harmful or threatening to your religious or spiritual beliefs. They are simply tools for tuning into higher consciousness, and have been utilized throughout the ages by everyone from Moses to Mohammed.

Meditation

Meditation is an attempt to attain some degree of mastery over the scattered thought processes of our minds. The Hindus and Buddhists like to compare our minds to "monkey minds." That's because, like monkeys our minds just love to chatter, ceaselessly switching from one subject to another.

Quieting the mind is the goal of meditation. As God says in the Bible, "Be still and know that I am God." It is in the quiet that God speaks to each one of us.

One school of meditation requires that you empty your mind of all these busy thoughts. Another school practices meditation by concentrating on one specific issue or problem in your life, such as what is at the root of my disease?

Another way of meditating requires that you employ all your meditative skills to make a meaningful connection with a symbol, such as one of the ten spheres located on the Tree of Life. In this technique, you concentrate on what that symbol means to you.

The Baal Shem Tov, the founder of Hassidism and a great practitioner of meditation, taught his own form of meditation. For this remarkable rabbi and Kabbalistic master, meditation did not mean just sitting down and spending from five minutes to an hour in mental solitude.

Instead, it meant to dwell *constantly* on one's thoughts of God's love for humankind. The Baal Shem Tov taught that even when washing dishes or conducting business you should be in meditation and thinking about God.

The rabbi would explain that even when doing business, you should not be thinking about how to be victorious over a competitor. Instead, your thoughts should be on how the two of you can both profit from this transaction. This, he said, was being in God consciousness.

Meditation becomes totally meaningless if it is not connected to your daily activities. You need to make all of your life a meditation by remaining aware of God's presence within and without. If you start separating things into "this is meditation" and "this is business," then you are not being a spiritual person.

I believe the most important thing about meditation is that it allows us the opportunity to hear our souls speaking to us. And because I am convinced that most physical, emotional, and mental illness stems from illnesses of the soul, we need to listen to that voice, and not just pay attention to our minds and bodies.

Meditation is an excellent way to tune into the spiritual presence within you. It is an invaluable tool in spiritual healing, one which offers therapeutic psychological and physical benefits, including greater self-awareness and personal transformation.

The meditations that appear throughout this book are all designed to help you to promote personal healing and well-being, and to enable you to tune into Divine guidance. Practice the meditations for at least ten minutes. Eventually, you can work your way up to thirty minutes of silent meditation.

Remember, no meditation is ever perfect. So, if in the course of your meditation, extraneous thoughts begin to slip into your mind—"I'm hungry," "I forgot to feed the cat," etcetera—simply acknowledge them with love in your heart and let them go. Except for perfect masters, these distractions plague all of us.

Remember not to get angry when your thoughts interrupt your meditation. Thoughts are living energies, which are also part of who you are. Let them pass with your blessings and then resume your meditation.

I predict that some of you are going to enjoy meditating so much that you will go overboard with it. Be careful of such a mind trap. Let me give you an example of how that trap can work.

Suppose a person spends a thousand dollars to study transcendental meditation. He comes home and he says to his family, "I got it now.

From now on, every morning, I'm going to get up at 6:00 A.M., wash up, and from 6:30 to 7:30 A.M. I'm going to meditate. I don't want anybody to interrupt me."

He practices his meditation for a week, two weeks, three weeks. One day, instead of getting up at 6:00 A.M. he gets up at 7:00 A.M. Now he wants to get washed up but the family is there—they have to go to work.

He grows angry and annoyed. "Don't you know I have to meditate," he shouts. "I'm already late. Get out of my way." Then he meditates for two hours and he's still angry that his schedule was thrown off.

He slams the door, turns down his wife's invitation to have breakfast with her and, while walking to work and at his business, he exhibits a bad temper all day. Was he truly meditating?

If he was truly meditating, the story would have gone this way:

He woke up late and he was angry, because we're only human. Then he goes to meditate. During his meditation he comes to realize how terribly he has treated his family. So the minute he gets through with his meditation, he apologizes to them. He embraces them and kisses them.

On the way to work he says hello to everybody. When a beggar stops him he gives him a dollar. At the office he creates heaven instead of hell.

That to me is meditation. You are more joyous and more charitable, and you see people and the world in a more positive sense.

Visualization

Visualization is another technique that we will employ throughout this book. This is a practice that uses the imagination to guide the body in a pleasurable, positive direction.

It is different from meditation because, instead of clearing the mind, you try to fill your mind with a strong image of what you desire. You are placing your conscious energy into that image, whether it be renewed health, more money, a new job, or a soulmate. You picture it as if it was already happening.

This is a powerful way of using thought forms to create energy and, believe it or not, it often works, depending on your powers of faith and concentration. I often practice such "seeing."

I like to visualize something from the world of matter, such as a tree or a blade of grass. I hold that picture in my mind's eye. And then, in my visualization, I look deeply into that tree or flower or blade of grass. I often see a spiritual form, which I recognize as a manifestation of God.

This practice helps me in my everyday life to see past the matter that constitutes a form (mineral, plant, animal, or human) and, instead, to see the spirit soul that each of us carries within. It helps me love all creatures who walk this earth.

Affirmation

An affirmation is a positive statement spoken as if something is already a reality. You are enforcing, or "making firm," that which you are imagining.

An example of an affirmation used in this book is *Lo amut*. In Hebrew, it means "I shall not die." Another affirmation is *Hakol beseder b'ezrath Hashem*, which translates as "All is in divine order with the help of God."

These are powerful statements, which, when spoken with confidence, can replace your weary and worn-out state of mind with positive ideas. Combined with a visualization, affirmations can, in a short period of time, bring about positive mental attitudes that can lead to healing.

The Tree of Life itself is an affirmation because it is perfect and expresses our own individual perfection. *I am the Tree of Life* is a good affirmation to repeat when you are feeling weak and uncertain.

For maintaining good health, I believe that you should begin each day with an affirmation, which expresses gratitude. After all, this is a day that God created for you, for me, for all of humanity.

An affirmation will help to make it a better day than yesterday. It will make it a more peaceful day, a more glorious day, a more joyful day. If you are ill, an affirmation can make it a hopeful day, a day in which God will work with you to improve your health.

One of my favorite morning affirmations is: *I am grateful to Thee, O Lord, for life*. Spoken in a powerful and convincing manner, it sets the stage for you to have a positive and purposeful day.

Choose any affirmation that makes you feel good about yourself and life. Two excellent affirmations you may choose to repeat if you are not feeling well are: *There is always a new beginning,* or *we are safe in the universe no matter what consequences ensue.*

Prayer

Prayer helps us to bring our individual consciousness into alignment with the universe and our highest spiritual realizations.

We will be talking more about prayer later on in this book. For the moment, keep in mind that during the act of prayer we are praising God and, in return, are usually asking for forgiveness or a favor. It is during such moments that we turn our heart toward God. We talk to God.

While in meditation, we try to listen to that still small voice. But during prayer we realize before whom we stand and ask for His/Her mercy and assistance.

Prayer, meditation, and visualization elicit a relaxation response in the mind. All these practices also help to hone the intuitive faculties, which are inherent in all of us, but are often neglected, much to our detriment.

To successfully travel the Tree of Life and to benefit from its healing powers, you must learn to rely on intuition and leave logic behind. Only then will you be able to taste the fruits of knowledge and wisdom that this magical tree has to offer you.

Introduction
What Is Kabbalah?

*"Eternal truths, eternal values, significant experiences
and genuine blessings like love, compassion, justice,
brotherhood, peace, and joy are to be found, not in
anything that can be measured, weighed, or counted,
but in that which is hidden from the eye."*
—Rabbi Isaac Luria, 16th Century Kabbalist—

"Everything that is visible, has an invisible part."
—Rainer Maria Rilke—

As you begin to read this book, the first question you might ask is, what does the word "Kabbalah" mean? It is an ancient Hebrew word which means "to receive," or "to reveal." So you might say that Kabbalah is a philosophy which reveals the mystical to the human mind.

The teachings of the Kabbalah do not stand alone. They are inextricably bound to the *Torah*, the first five books of the Old Testament. But the language of the Kabbalah is much more mystical and abstract than its companion work. The *Torah* is the heart of Wisdom while the Kabbalah can be considered its soul.

The Tree of Life is the primary symbol of Kabbalah. It is a diagram containing ten *sefiroth*—also called spheres or globes—and various paths. These spheres are believed to contain clues to the mysteries and meaning of life (see Fig. 1).

Each of these spheres represents an aspect of the Divine and, since as Kabbalists believe we are part of the Divine, then these symbols correspond to attributes within ourselves as well.

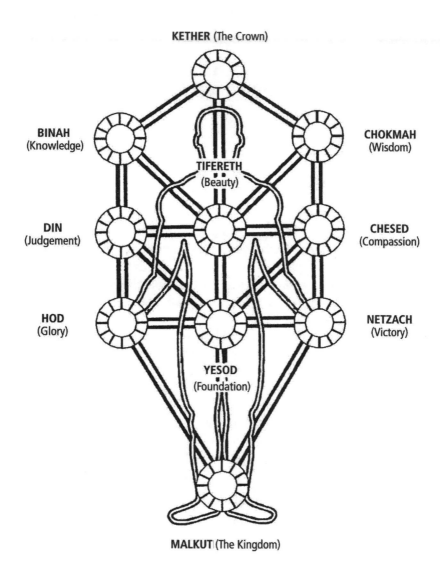

KETHER (The Crown)

BINAH
(Knowledge)

CHOKMAH
(Wisdom)

TIFERETH
(Beauty)

DIN
(Judgement)

CHESED
(Compassion)

HOD
(Glory)

NETZACH
(Victory)

YESOD
(Foundation)

MALKUT (The Kingdom)

Figure 1: Tree of Life

Much has been written about this sacred tree over the centuries. Mystics have described it as everything from a "cosmic map of consciousness" to the key to astrology, numerology, tarot, and angel lore.

All the above may be true. But for the purposes of this book it is important for you to know that the Tree of Life is essentially a potent psychological tool for self-discovery and profound inner knowing—one which can lead to health, happiness, harmony, and joy.

Despite its many revelatory teachings, the teachings of Kabbalah have not always been eagerly accepted. Even today I'm not certain that we are truly ready to receive this secret knowledge completely.

In Hassidic literature, there is even a story about our reluctance to embrace Kabbalah. The setting for this tale is the foot of Mount Sinai, where God supposedly first tried to explain this mystical system to the Israelites who were gathered there.

According to the tradition, instead of eagerly accepting these revelations, the Israelites balked and practically fainted from the ecstasy brought on by this communication. They ran from the mountain and formed a committee to speak to Moses.

The leader of the committee asked Moses to tell God not to continue speaking to the people about such things. "We are not ready!" the spokesman complained. "You continue for us. You're already accustomed to it."

So, many thousands of years ago humankind missed a tremendous opportunity to receive the secrets of the Kabbalah directly from its source. We were not ready. As a result, Kabbalah was left out of the common teachings and was shared only by the selected elders of Israel.

Nonetheless, Kabbalah has survived and remains one of the oldest systems of mystical thought available to us today. It concerns itself with the mysteries of body, mind, and soul. It guides us along spiritual paths towards wholeness. It shows us how to live a healthy, joyful, balanced, and meaningful life.

The earliest known mention of Kabbalah is the use of the word *Merkabah*—the Throne—by Ezekiel. The throne represents the sphere which appears at the top of the Tree of Life. The image of such a "mystic throne" also appears in Kabbalistic literature during the second century in Palestine.

Mystical tradition holds that God was the first Kabbalist, and that He/She imparted that knowledge to Adam in the Garden of Eden. God later revealed Kabbalah to Abraham, Noah, and Moses.

A historical explanation suggests that Kabbalah's two main bodies of work, the *Sepher Yetzereh*, or *Book of Formation* and the *Zohar*, or the

Book of Splendour, were written respectively in the second century A.D and thirteenth century Spain.

The *Sepher Yetzereh* was supposedly written by the enlightened Jewish mystic, Rabbi Akiba, or by Akiba's disciple, Rabbi Simon Ben Yohai. This was an era when the Jews were under Roman oppression and were seeking some metaphysical solace from their tyranny.

Whatever the origin of these works, their teachings were secretly preserved by Jewish mystics who devoted their lives to their study and passed these secrets down from generation to generation.

Every generation has had its Kabbalists who pondered the mysteries of these ancient texts—often while in hiding. Each generation had its teachers, the ones chosen to share a part of these divine revelations with others.

I believe I was chosen to teach Kabbalah in this generation. In fact, I feel a very strong connection to Rabbi Shimon Ben Yohai, one of the authors of the Kabbalah. I believe I may be the reincarnated soul of one of his students who, fearful of Roman persecution, hid in a cave with the rabbi outside Jerusalem where they discussed the mysteries of this great work.

Yes, I do believe in reincarnation. Can one learn in just one lifetime all one needs to learn in order to cleave unto the Lord? I don't think so. To grow in spiritual understanding through each lifetime is the voyage and real purpose of life.

Some readers may worry that a study of Kabbalah will compromise their religious beliefs. Fear not! The Kabbalah is not an object of worship and it does not represent any one religion. It is a path to awakening and self-discovery which reveals universal truths that are at the core of all religions.

Kabbalah got a boost in thirteenth century Spain, when there was a revival of interest in these esoteric writings. Suddenly, this hidden knowledge became popularized.

Towards the end of that century a Spanish rabbi by the name of Moses de Leon wrote a kind of mystery novel about Kabbalah. This work was called the *Zohar,* and its teachings became widely available to Christians and Jews alike.

The Kabbalah, which originally was a purely devotional system that focused upon the ten divine attributes of God, began to be applied in practical ways for improving spiritual, physical, mental, and emotional health. Later, it became the basis for the Western mystery tradition.

It is a metaphysical system that has had a profound influence on everyone from Jesus and the Essenes to Madame Blavatsky, the founder of Theosophy. In fact, much of her "Secret Doctrine" was essentially composed of Kabbalistic ideas.

Kabbalah is vast in its teachings. It makes use of numbers (gematria), and sacred letters of the Hebrew alphabet as part of its reservoir of hidden knowledge.

But despite all that, the study of Kabbalah is not really that complicated. Let me reassure you that there is nothing in this system which is so mystical that you or I couldn't understand it. As Isaac said in the Bible, "What we seek is merely hidden from our physical eyes."

All we need is the third eye—the eye of spirit—to see it. With such spiritual eyes, Kabbalah is crystal clear.

For example, suppose you've lost a diamond in a dark room. You know it's there but you can't see it. Now suppose someone hands you a bright flashlight. With its intense light you can easily see the diamond, because it was there all along. Consider this book your spiritual flashlight.

By the time you have finished reading this book, not only will you have grasped the essentials of Kabbalism, but you will also be able to apply it to your healing work.

Think of these "essentials" as the nine rungs on a ladder leading upward toward God consciousness. These rungs are:

1. To be one with the self, the soul, and *Shekinah*—God's indwelling feminine presence.
2. To forgive the past and look forward to the future with joy and excitement.
3. To open the mind, letting the soul fly into unknown space.
4. To be aware of the Ten Emanations of God—symbolized by the Tree of Life—that interact within each of us.
5. To consider what our true mission in life is, and to be totally alive to that mission.

6. To be ready once again to hear the message given at Mount Sinai to love thy neighbor as thyself.
7. To learn the art and science of living spiritually—healthy in body, mind, and soul.
8. To experience genuine love and know the difference between pleasure, happiness, and joy.
9. To reunite the divided self in order to know the glory of the oneness of God.

One of Kabbalah's most important concepts is that without human effort, God will remain unredeemed. God only lives where He/She is invited. In other words, we are responsible for God's intervention on earth.

If you want God in your life to help you improve or maintain your health or for any other reason, all you need to do is call. This is one of the important keys to the understanding of Kabbalah. There is an interactive arrangement between God and yourself, a partnership, so to speak.

One of my favorite actresses, Elizabeth Taylor, a longtime devotee of Kabbalah, recently offered her own interpretation of this mystical work. When interviewed while in a wheelchair because of a broken back, she said:

"Through my studies I'm able to see how everything happens for a reason. Pain comes to us all to teach us life lessons, to focus our souls on what's precious in life. Through Kabbalah, I feel empowered like never before to work through my physical ailments."

It's a wonderful explanation. If you were to ask me in one sentence what the Kabbalah teaches, it is what the Baal Shem Tov suggested: "The greatest sin is having a melancholic attitude, to worry, or to be depressed." Miss Taylor certainly wasn't having any such feelings during her painful ordeal.

So, finally, what is Kabbalah? As I see it, it is the face of God extoling us to make His/Her hidden light shine in our daily relationships and experiences. It is the ultimate meaning of existence.

Kabbalah is about a spiritual quest, one which you are soon to embark upon. It is a quest for true knowledge and understanding that will lead you to explore the very depths of your heart and soul in order to receive God's healing grace.

A Partnership with God

"Walk humbly with God as an equal."
—The Prophet Micah—

We all have problems. Life is not always good or peaceful or joyous. We are not finished creatures and have much to do if we are to attain a state of perfection.

During a deep state of meditation I had a vision that I would like to share with you. I saw the Creator inviting Adam and Eve to tea. And God said to them: "Let me tell you what I did during the last six days.

> On the first day I created the eternal light. On the second day I separated the waters above and below, so that the Earth was visible. On the third day I created nature, the trees, the flowers, grass, and on the fourth day I created the heavenly bodies, the sun, the moon, and the stars.
>
> On the fifth day I created most of the animals, and today I created you—Adam and Eve. And I want to tell you something. From now on I won't do anything by myself. You and I together will finish the creation.

That work and that partnership are still in effect. Until it is completed—until we human beings reach a stage of perfection that will satisfy the Creator—our imperfections will continue. And one of those imperfections is our vulnerability to illness and disease.

Perhaps the most important point of this anecdote is that we are partners with God. Among the ancient mystics this partnership was known as *Shutaf Elohim.*

The early Kabbalists had a universal vision that compelled them to see the presence of God in all beings. They lived their lives with this partnership always in mind.

The Bible says that God created man and then woman because the Creator believed "it was not good for man to be alone." The Kabbalists focused on this statement and explained that God knew the pain of loneliness. God was alone before He/She created the first human creatures.

So God created Adam and Eve. He also created partners among the days. Monday has Sunday, Wednesday has Tuesday, Friday has Thursday, and Saturday has God.

This concept of a divine/human partnership is an important point for you to remember whether or not you are in need of healing. You must always remember that there is nothing that God can do without us, and there is nothing anyone can do without God.

God needs us as much as we need God. So the Creator is always available for help and support each time you call upon Him/Her. After all, what else are partners for? And for this partnership to work, God needs us to be well. If you are sick, God is sick. Which is why the Lord has a vested interest in keeping us healthy. Because we are partners with God, we must take the personal responsibility to work with Him/Her and complete ourselves, and that includes times when we are not feeling well.

Do you know the Hebrew blessing over bread? "Praise be the Lord for bringing forth bread from the earth." What does it mean that God is bringing forth bread? I believe this blessing is a reminder that before we were created the Lord did everything by Himself/Herself. But after man was created, God said "from now on you have to help me plan for the future in order to survive."

My understanding of the blessing over bread came to me in a dream during *Rosh Hashona*, the Jewish New Year.

In that dream I heard the word *barach*, which means "blessed be." And I said, "blessed be who?" And the answer came back, "You." I said, "who's this talking?" The voice said "Your God, King of the Universe."

I said, "Yes, what do you want?" The Almighty then explained the prayer over bread to me. God said that it should be translated as "*You* bring forth bread from the earth." You do it and make it happen through your efforts—planting, cultivating, and harvesting the grain. That's part of the Divine/human partnership.

Basically the Kabbalah teaches us that our mission on earth is to be in partnership with God. The Almighty did His/Her part, and now you do your part.

Your part is to remain awake to and aware of your special relationship with the Lord. There's nothing separate between the two of you. It is *always* the two of you together. *Shutaf Elohim.*

Being Awake and Aware

To be awake and aware are the two most important concepts for you to understand in your quest to maintain or repair your health. You must become alert to the fact that your kingdom—your body—is your responsibility.

In addition, you must also become aware that it is okay to call upon your partner God for help, if you need help. We're all connected, anyway. The physical body is connected to the spiritual and emotional bodies, and everything is connected to God.

In Jeremiah 17 we read about the importance of such awareness. The prophet says that "the cursed man shall not see when good cometh." What Jeremiah is saying is that God is constantly doing good for you, but you lose if you are not receptive to the signs.

Another story emphasizing the importance of awareness involves the Buddha, who was once asked, "Who are you? Are you God?" Buddha said, "No." "Are you a son of God?" He said, "No. I'm not."

Then he was asked, "Are you a saint or a holy man?" Again, the Buddha replied that he was not. "Then what are you?" the questioner asked. "I am awake," Buddha replied. "I am aware of all the nuances in life and I am aware as I look at every human being of seeing the image of God in him."

Awareness and awakefulness are the two most important words to remember if you want to be fully alive and healthy or effect your own or someone else's healing. You must remain aware of the oneness of everything, the connectedness of everything.

You must become aware of the *Shekinah*, the female divinity, as well as the *Neshama*, which means "soul" in Hebrew. These feminine principles, which we will talk about in more detail later in this book, can be very helpful in preserving or repairing health.

Like Buddha, the Kabbalists have been practicing their version of awareness for hundreds of years. These ancient mystics called it *kavanna,* or concentrated awareness.

In Kabbalistic literature, there are many accounts of how these mystics attained such a state of awareness. When they awoke in the morning and before they fell asleep at night they would concentrate on *kavanah,* and express gratefulness for the miracle of God's presence in their lives.

When I arise each morning, and before I fall asleep, I experience the awareness of God's presence within me, and along with that experience of knowingness, comes a feeling of gratefulness.

You should practice *kavanah*—awareness of God—and awareness of the *Shekinah* and the soul whenever possible whether you are feeling well or ill. It will help put you into a frame of mind that is conducive to healing.

Sometimes when I am teaching my Kabbalah students about the ways in which we are all one—even with that homeless person sleeping on the street—and the need to be awake to that fact, I will walk over to one of my pupils and I step on his or her toe.

They'll jump up and say, "What happened? You just stepped on my toe." I say, "How many toes do you have?" They'll say, "ten." Then I ask, "When was the last time you counted them? When was the last time you thought of that little toe?"

I stepped on that little toe to remind my student that it was connected to the other nine toes, and that those ten toes were connected to his feet, his feet to his ankle, his ankle to his leg, and so on.

The little toe represents everyone we don't really think about; the homeless, the poor, the ill, the starving Africans, the Chinese peasants and, in some cases, even our partner God.

And unless you're awake to this totally, unless you're aware that all of mankind is one and that we are connected to God who is also One, then we're a divided and ineffectual self.

Healing does not come from division of body, mind, and soul, but from integration of all these aspects of our body and senses. Health is wholeness and wholeness is health. And wholeness comes from an awareness that we are in partnership with God.

Purpose

I think "Thou Shalt Have Purpose" should be the Eleventh Commandment, because this concept is so important for healing and living life to its fullest.

Having purpose means possessing the ability to say "yes" to life—to be in love with life. A sense of purpose is also a vital element in strengthening your partnership with God. Certainly, it's nice to be in business with the Creator, but what is the purpose of your work?

If you are ill, your purpose should be getting well. If you are not sick, your purpose should be staying healthy. Many people who are ill say they want to get well, but don't really mean it. There's no real purpose behind their words.

Some people prefer *kvetching*—or complaining—to healing. They have lost their purpose—which is recovery. Instead, they seem to pride themselves on being sick. People often tell me, "I'm sicker than you," or "I've been in therapy for ten years. I'm really sick."

This is not purposeful thinking. It's a kind of negativism. To have purpose means to be inspired to respond to the challenges of ill health, to say "I am" and "I will be." It means being awake and aware of opportunities to improve your health. It means feeling the spirit of God within you.

A purposeful individual will rally and respond to his or her physical or emotional challenge, while a less purposeful person will either continue to *kvetch* about it or decide to live a life filled with frustration and anxiety. So which one are you? A *kvetcher* or a doer?

Possibly, one reason you decided to purchase this particular book is because you thought that by reading it you might learn something about how Kabbalah can be used for promoting good health.

That's a good example of purposeful thinking. You want to complete something, which, if you are ill, is the restoration of your health. In Genesis, Chapter 11, it is written: "And God blessed the seventh day and hallowed it, because on that day He rested from all His work, which God created to make."

Notice the words—"which God created to make" or "*la'asot*" in Hebrew. This can be interpreted as the purpose of man is to help God to finish creation or, in your case, to have God help you complete your healing.

God did not complete creation. He/She purposely assigned man the task of completing it. He wanted to give man (and woman) purpose. Is that what you are doing right now by reading this book, being purposeful? If it is, never let go of that attitude. Always remember that you are the co-creator of your health. You are *Shutaf Elohim*, in partnership with God.

You also have purpose when you decide to be "fully alive" despite your illness; when you don't allow disease to crush you and turn you into a creature of melancholy and despair.

You manifest purpose when, instead of wallowing in negative emotions, you put all your intuitive and intellectual skills to work for healing.

Remember that God has created you with all the wisdom and ability and awareness that you need to purposefully carry on with your life. Do your best and the best will come back to you. God created you to be healthy, not sick. Your purpose is to work with God to restore your damaged health.

Whenever you are feeling down or depressed, repeating the following affirmation may help lift your spirits. It will remind you of your special relationship with your Creator:

> *O my God, perfection is my aim and my aim is perfect. For I have purpose. The spirit of God guides me graciously and lovingly in all the steps of this attainment. Divine Mind, assure my success, for I have purpose.*

Staying Balanced

Any effective partnership is an exercise in balance leading to purposeful activity. We learn the strengths and weaknesses of our partner and once we understand the dynamics of our relationship, we are able to work more purposefully to create something positive.

The Kabbalistic Tree of Life also speaks of balance. Looking at a diagram of the sacred tree you will notice that there are ten spheres. Three on the right side, three on the left, and four down the middle "trunk."

Despite the fact that these spheres are directly linked to each other

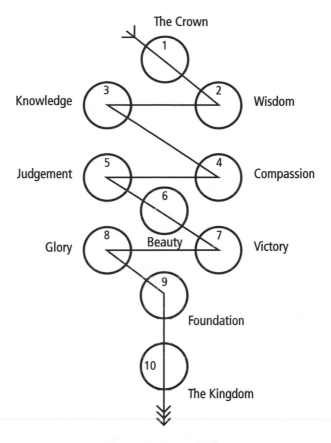

Figure 2: Tree of Life

by the "branches," or paths, of the tree, each of these spheres has characteristics that are often in dynamic opposition to each other.

For example, the sphere of Wisdom is directly linked to the sphere of Knowledge. According to Kabbalah, Wisdom and Knowledge are considered opposites of each other. Wisdom represents purpose and spiritual will, while knowledge corresponds to understanding, awareness, and spiritual love.

Similarly, the sphere of Compassion is connected to that of Judgment. These two globes are also dynamically opposed. Compassion corresponds to mercy, while Judgment has a strong feeling of severity attached to it.

A bit lower down on the tree, the sphere of Victory is connected to Glory. These two globes are also in dynamic opposition to each other.

While Victory often symbolizes ego and our carnal side, Glory in Splendour deals with issues relating to humility and the mastery of our baser nature.

Despite such opposing qualities, all these spheres are nonetheless in equilibrium. That's because, according to Kabbalah, equilibrium or balance results from harmonizing opposing forces.

For example, most of us think of ourselves as a single identity, but what appears to be a single identity is a body with many opposing characteristics such as good and evil, innocence and guile, yin and yang.

We are part this and part that, part masculine and part feminine. All these opposing parts do not make us fragmented personalities unless one of our aspects becomes unbalanced and upsets our equilibrium. Then we can become a Hitler or a Hannibal Lechter. Otherwise we remain in harmony.

In fact, according to Kabbalah, such opposing tendencies play an important role in both our spiritual growth and in strengthening and protecting us.

Kabbalists believe spiritual growth is promoted when we become aware of these divergent energies and strive to keep them in balance. They further believe that our positive inclinations or impulses, *yetzer hatov*, are balanced by our negative inclinations, *yetzer harah*, and the combination of these polarities empower us.

According to Kabbalistic tradition, our positive impulses are represented by the right arm and fingers of the right hand. This corresponds to the right side of the Tree of Life. Our negative impulses are represented by the left arm and fingers, corresponding to the sacred tree's left side.

In my Hassidic tradition, as well as in Christian theology, we are taught that any negativity must be eliminated. So if I followed either of these traditions to the letter of the law, I would have to think about cutting off my left arm to get rid of the negative impulses.

But Kabbalists believe that anything that is alive—and that includes negative thoughts or feelings—should never be killed but, instead, harmonized. Rather than kill negativity, isn't it be better to combine it with positive thinking and thus create a new life called harmony? Not only would I be refining any negativity, but the combination of these two potent forces would actually make me a stronger person. I would have balanced one strong power with another. Even more importantly, I would not have to live my life as a one-armed cripple.

It is by maintaining balance that you are both strengthened and protected. There was no need to cut off your left arm, which would have created imbalance. Certainly such drastic action would remove the symptom of negativity, but it would cause big physical problems down the line.

Dis-ease means not being at ease with yourself—feeling out of balance. Unless you recognize the importance of maintaining a harmonious interplay between mind, body, and soul, you can do harm to your physical or emotional health.

Another lesson that illustrates the importance of balance is the "Star of David," which is a Kabbalistic Symbol. This so-called "Jewish star" is made up of two triangles—one pointing to heaven and, the other pointing to earth. These two triangles symbolize perfect balance.

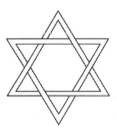

Figure 3: Star of David

Please note that "Star of David" is not an accurate translation of the Hebrew word, *Mogen David,* which actually means the "Shield of David." Shield of David makes more sense, because it refers to King David, who was not only a poet and the author of the Psalms, but also a warrior.

When at war, he carried his unique shield before him to protect his heart from arrows. He believed that this symbol of the two triangles had power because it was a union of opposites. Balance protected him.

So if you are ill, or experiencing sorrow rather than joy, try to balance those feelings by looking at the other side of the coin. This is the time to mobilize a different inner perspective.

For example, you might think of your illness as a growth experience rather than a total catastrophe. There may be important lessons that you need to learn in this lifetime before moving on to the next, and illness might afford you the opportunity to slow down and reconsider your purpose in life.

In fact, I tend to believe that the cause of many illnesses is that for too long we have neglected our souls. If I am correct, perhaps this is the deeper reason for the onset of your disease. You may be spiritually out of balance. Think about that possibility and try to make adjustments. Awareness of the spiritual aspects of illness can lead to true healing.

I had a client who lived a lifestyle in which spirituality played almost no role. Katy was an attractive young woman who drank alcohol excessively and generally had a poor diet. She was completely out of balance in body, mind, and soul.

It was only when she was diagnosed with a serious disease that Katy, for the first time in her life, became interested in spiritual matters. She also began to develop a real sense of purpose.

This young woman geared up to fight her disease, despite the pessimistic views of her doctor that chances of improvement were slim. In addition to reading spiritual literature, Katy now began to devour books written by alternative health experts such as Gary Null and Dr. Andrew Weil.

She also began to meditate, practiced yoga, and substituted green tea and wheat grass for alcohol. French fries were replaced by brown rice, and Katy started a macrobiotic diet. Friday night was no longer reserved for renting movies or sitting in a bar, but for religious services.

It was her disease that started Katy along this road. For the first time in years, she began to pay attention to her body, mind, and soul. And within two years her condition had improved so much that even her doctor was amazed at her progress.

Today, Katy continues to heal. She has not abandoned her new, more positive lifestyle. Illness turned her into a co-creator with the Great Architect of life, and I believe that if this young woman continues on this path, she will one day completely recover.

Avoiding Imbalance

Our balance can be upset by many things, among them fear, anger, hostility, eating poorly, not exercising regularly, a judgmental attitude, carnal behavior, and spiritual bankruptcy.

If you work out in the gym seven days a week and fail to exercise your spiritual muscles even once a week, then you are out of balance.

If, on the other hand, you do nothing but engage in spiritual activities and stay away from the gym, you are also out of balance. If you get plenty of exercise and are a regular churchgoer but don't exercise your mind, you are not in balance.

Any of these imbalances can eventually lead to some kind of distress. We know that the day is reserved for work, the night is for rest, and that the body needs to be fed. But then what about the soul? What are you doing for her? This is another example of poor equilibrium.

A personal story illustrates the importance of balance. I was about eleven years old and living in a small Hungarian village. One night, in the middle of the night, I knocked on the door of my father's room. I said, "I can't sleep."

My father said, "Did you say your evening prayers?" I said, "No, I forgot." I said my prayers and was able to go to sleep. You see, the soul was accustomed to hearing these prayers. She didn't hear them so she wouldn't let me sleep. She was out of balance.

The soul is usually very quiet. But this evening she spoke up. She said, "Hey, you did something wrong." She pointed out that her body was satisfied because she had walked a long way during the day, and her mind was satisfied because she had read a newspaper before she went to bed. But, she said "I had done nothing for my soul. My soul scolded me because I had neglected her. I had thrown myself out of balance."

You must learn to avoid imbalances in order to maintain or regain good health. You must nurture your body as well as your emotional, intellectual, and spiritual levels. You must grow simultaneously on *all* levels to become a healthy and mature person.

Spiritual Balance

I cannot overemphasize the importance of maintaining spiritual balance if you are truly interested in promoting good health. There are two ways to stay healthy. One way is not to get ill in the first place. The second way is to determine how to get rid of sickness once you are sick. Spirituality plays a key role in both these equations.

I believe that one way not to get ill is to remain in God consciousness. And that means finding out exactly what is it that God wants you to do today. That's what meditation is for; to listen and find out what God wants from you. This approach can lead to balance. It is an excellent way to listen to God who is constantly talking to us through our soul. The problem, of course, is that not many of us bother to listen.

The Kabbalah relates that when God appeared at Mount Sinai to give us the Ten Commandments, that was only *one* of many appearances. The mystics believed that the Creator has never stopped communicating with us.

Is it very important to listen. It is also good etiquette. We should try to listen not only to God, who always has healing words to offer us if we pay attention, but we should also learn to listen more to each other. Who knows what we can learn about what ails us from listening?

If you have fallen ill and are not a spiritual person, after first consulting with your doctor, you must try to attain a spiritual state of mind. You must try to connect with God. One simple way to do this is to feel grateful for every piece of bread that you eat and every sip of water that you drink.

Express gratitude for everything that you put in the body. This attitude of gratefulness will help you to restore your spiritual balance. Also, thank God for still being alive. Yes, you are sick, but you are still alive and things can always change overnight. Miracles can and do happen!

But miracles require faith. Faith means stepping boldly out of a known groove into a brand new channel, and doing so with eagerness rather than with trepidation. It means letting go of your negative companions, fear and futility.

Sri Swami Satchidananda said it best: "If you have total faith in a Higher Will—a Higher Energy—you will be able to tune into that and receive all the strength and energy to recharge your system."

To attain spiritual balance, it is also helpful to occupy your mind with thoughts that are not about your symptoms. Read stories of human kindness, or inspiring stories about joy and peace.

Books about people who conquered their own illnesses are also important to read. The Bible is a wonderful book that is filled with inspirational stories of miraculous healings.

Reading biographies can be helpful as well. Most great people had to conquer something in their lives—either some sickness or an attitude that held them back—to become the great people that they were. Reading such stories will help you to open your spiritual eyes.

Another excellent way to attain a spiritual state of mind is by meditating on the Tree of Life, which you will learn later on in this book. It will not only help you to establish an awareness of spirituality in your life, but also show you how to "tune into" the possible root causes of your illness.

Finding out "how come?" is always a good pursuit when you are trying to recover from an illness. The first question that many Native American shamans ask is "Why?" What is the spiritual cause for this illness? "Why" is always the question that holds the key to the answers you seek.

Choose Life

Day has a night, and life has joy and sorrow, sickness and health. There is darkness and light, good and bad, beauty and ugliness. Finding meaning is the adventure, the challenge, the excitement. But this can only be undertaken when we affirm that "to live is the rarest thing in the world." Making life meaningful demands focusing on the *me* in meaningful and the *make* in making.

According to Kabbalah, there are seven opposites. They are: grace/sin; knowledge/ignorance; wealth/poverty; power/slavery; fertility/sterility; peace/war; life/death. I like to throw in an extra: sorrow/joy.

I like to finish with joy because it is based on the Biblical recommendation by Moses, our teacher, bless his soul, who mentioned it to his people when he was planning to depart from them forever. He said, "I've spoken to you about the curse and the blessings. Didn't I? And I've spoken to you about life and death. Didn't I? Now it's your choice. Choose." And then he added these beautiful words: "And I beg you to choose life."

Exercise

Stand up and take your right arm—the one that represents your good inclinations—and swing it to the left side of your body at waist level. Now, take your left arm—the one that represents your negative inclinations—and swing it at waist level to the right side of your body. Repeat this swinging gesture two or three times. By doing so you are creating balance.

Next, take your right hand and place it on your left shoulder—positive on negative. Reverse this movement. Left hand on right shoulder. Do this ten times as you visualize balance being restored in your body and God's grace coming through the top of your head in healing white light. This is where the *Shekinah* enters our bodies.

Now visualize angels coming through a portal at the top of your head and imbuing you with joy and the light of grace. Also think of negative things you wish to get rid of: Disease, sin, poverty, melancholy, pessimism, et cetera.

Next, raise your hands palms up and look at your fingers. Let each finger represent something you want to get rid of. Maybe it's bad health, or poverty, or fear. Perhaps it's some sin you committed during the week, war in the world, or an end to homelessness. Shake off all these negative attributes. Let them be gone from you!

Now visualize your ten fingers as candles. They are burning with joy and health and peace of mind. Affirm that healing is coming into your life. In your mind's eye, see yourself as perfectly healthy.

Choose life, choose love, and get ready to live! Now, say: *Hakol baseder b'ezrat Hashem.* All is in divine order with the help of God.

The Tyranny of Fear

"It is not death or hardship that is a fearful thing,
but the fear of hardship and death."
—Epictetus—

Not only must you maintain balance for optimal health, but you must also do your utmost to eliminate fear. Fear is a tyrant that holds good health in hostage.

It's easy to feel fear when you are sick. Am I going to die? Will I lose my job? How will I pay my bills? Who will support my family? Such fears plague all of us when we are in the grip of some disease.

But fear is only a tyrant that is empowered by permission. We are the ones who open the door and let it slip in. It thrives and grows and eliminates the space we need to live life to its fullest.

I believe that the cause of any sickness not only is connected to the soul, but also is connected with the mind. Why am I sick? Because I think I am sick. Maybe I'm not really sick, but my mind says that I am. Fear can often make us think this way.

Basically, we hurt ourselves, and can cause great damage to our bodies, when we permit fear to take over. We're all vulnerable to fear.

Recently, when I had a little cold, I experienced some fear. I thought, "What if I get pneumonia?" This is a human reaction. But then I caught myself. I thought, "No, I'm not getting ill." And eventually the cold passed without any other harmful effects.

We must try to be mindful of the crippling and negative effects of fear and try to put it aside. One excellent way to do this is by reading spiritual literature. You might also try visualizing positive objects like the crucifix, Torah, or even the image of the Tree of Life. All of these images contain within them the power to protect you from harm.

Fear is one way Satan tries to make us feel alone and separate us from God and our fellow human beings. By visualizing holy objects, you are staying connected to God.

Positive action also helps. Something as simple as arguing with God is an example of such action. Whenever I'm feeling ill I argue with God. It helps me replace my fear with some positive activity. It puts my mind somewhere else. I clasp my fists, raise my hands, and go through all the motions of someone involved in a good argument. I tell God that I want Him/Her to get rid of my illness. I ask how I can serve God if I'm not feeling well?

There is absolutely nothing wrong with arguing with God. It's a good release, and God certainly doesn't mind.

This is similar to two people in a relationship. They can argue, but it doesn't mean that they don't love each other. As a matter of fact, if there are no arguments in a relationship, I wonder if these people do love each other.

This reminds me of a story about a rabbi who, on *Yom Kippur*, the holiest day in the Jewish calendar, got into an argument with God. The rabbi was opening the ark where the Torah is kept and was getting ready to begin his prayers. Suddenly he stopped. He said, "I want to talk to you, God. I have an argument with you. You're supposed to be compassionate, loving, omnipotent, but what kind of God are you? Just look at the world."

The rabbi went on to recite a litany of injustices from disease to the Holocaust. He spent an hour arguing with God. "Why don't you do something about all this?" he said. "I'm not leaving this synagogue until I hear an answer from you."

Long minutes passed and there was nothing but silence. The rabbi finally picked up his prayer book and began saying prayers to glorify and sanctify God. Even without an answer, the rabbi continued to believe in and praise the Lord.

Each morning I practice a Kabbalistic meditation that not only helps me to chase away my fears, but also to confirm life. It incorporates some physical movement. If your mornings are too busy to do this exercise, try it before you go to sleep.

Exercise

Find a quiet place in your home where you won't be disturbed by ringing telephones or anything else. Like King Solomon used to do during meditation and prayer, get down on your knees.

Raise your hands with palms facing up to the heavens. Choose a prayer from the back of this book—or one of your own—and repeat that prayer seven times. You may substitute one of God's Holy Names like *El Shadai* or *Yehovah* if you so choose.

Next, lay down on your stomach. This is a position of humility. It symbolizes the question: "Who Am I?" Place your outstretched hands palms down on the floor. Lift up your head and say: "*Ho du l'Adonai*," a Kabbalistic phrase meaning "Praise the Lord."

As you repeat this phrase, keep thinking: *I'm alive and I'm healthy. I have no fear because God is with me.* Then turn your head to the right and repeat three times: "*Ki Tov.*" It translates into "all is well," or "all is good."

Next, turn your head to the left and again repeat those words. "*Ki Tov.*"

Sit up and say, "*Ke l'olam Hasdo*"—the "whole world is filled with God's loving kindness." Visualize the whole world living in peace, harmony, and in good health. See yourself as part of that world feeling perfectly healthy.

Dethroning Fear

"Do not fear. Act!"
—Kabbalistic adage—

Fear not only holds health hostage, it is always hope's worst enemy. To dethrone fear you must replace "I cannot," with "I can." You must learn how to say with confidence and courage, "I can promote health."

To rid yourself of your fear you must try to replace it with joy and enthusiasm. In the one-hundredth Psalm, the Psalmist said: "Serve the Lord in gladness." The writer of this psalm used the word *simchah*, which in English can mean happiness.

It means more than that, it also means joy. You must be in the state of joy to truly serve the Lord. Fear robs us of that joy. So if you are not feeling well, accept that you may have to go to the doctor, but also try to balance any fear that you may be experiencing with joyful thoughts about the outcome of that doctor's visit.

You may wish to practice repeating one of the following affirmations: *"God is the only power and the only presence." "God is with me and I do not fear." "I anticipate all impending events with enthusiasm and expectations of good."*

Have complete faith that God will be there to help and guide you. For example, when I get sick I say to myself, "Oh, I'm sick," but I also quickly add, "Isn't that wonderful, I feel pain. It's a sign that I'm still alive. Only the dead feel no pain."

If on a day I feel ill someone asks me, "How do you feel?" I reply, "I'm okay, although I'm not feeling well." What I am doing is expressing faith that although I am not feeling well at the moment, with God's help, this too shall pass.

I also try to say to myself, "All right, this hurts and that hurts. Yesterday I was feeling all right and tomorrow maybe I'll be all right again."

This is another way that I try to eliminate fear from my life. I'm trying to dethrone a mental tyrant who, if I let it, will rule my life.

There is a Kabbalistic aphorism that you may wish to memorize: "When you are sick the whole world is sick—including God." And if God is not feeling well, you have a pretty powerful partner who is going to bat for your healing so that both of you can get back to work building His/Her kingdom on earth.

The best way to dethrone fear in order to promote health is to fill yourself with positive and loving thoughts of God. Suppose, for example, that you put a drop of ink in water. Immediately, the water becomes black. So how do you make the water return to its original clearness? You add a lot more water until the ink becomes dispersed.

If you are ill and feeling frightened, add a lot of positive imagery to your thinking and manner of speech. It will help to displace fear. One visualization technique I like to use when I'm not feeling well is to imagine a healthy new baby coming out of its mother's womb.

Or I try to visualize the spirit of God in me. If God is in you, how can you not be healthy? See God as light or energy, or use any other metaphor that denotes a spiritual presence.

However you choose to express it, the most important thing is to love God with all your heart and all your soul and all your might. Fear separates us from this kind of love. Pay attention to your thoughts and feelings so that you do not do some foolish thing that would be untrue to yourself and be a less than complete expression of your love for the Lord.

The Baal Shem Tov taught there was only one plan in life, to "live in joy!"—to live in the name of God. Fear short circuits that kind of thinking. It is something you cannot afford to do on your quest for health.

Melancholy

One of the most self-defeating forms of fear is melancholy. Melancholy weakens faith. It is a form of surrender. If you lift this veil of sadness and nurture life instead, you will learn how to participate in joy again.

You must eliminate melancholy from your life, and that can be done only by uniting with spirit—by being aware of your partnership with the Lord.

Remember that no person or circumstance can defeat you if you keep your channels open to God's healing spirit. Melancholy is negative thinking and blocks these channels. So live courageously, live calmly, live positively.

Anger

Anger is fear's partner and another enemy of true healing. In order to de-throne fear, we must also try to rid ourselves of anger. It is natural to feel anger when we feel sick, sad, or disappointed, but anger is poison. The more we take in the more we poison ourselves. Imagine that you are thirsty and I bring you a glass of water. Do you think you would drink the water if I told you I put some poison it. The minute you feel anger coming on become aware of it and say, "Oh, my God, I'm not drinking that water. It's poisoned." Then visualize the Tree of Life. Anger and hos-tility can create sickness in us, and fear can keep it there.

Anytime you feel angry—whether it is over your health problems or for any other reason—take some time off and pay a visit to the Tree of Life. When you are in the midst of your meditation on the tree, ask your-self "Why am I so angry?" and take a journey within.

Creating anger is not your mission in life, because it can express itself as illness. All anger really does is steal your freedom. Instead, ac-cept the adversity you may be experiencing, reject anger and defeat, and let those harmful emotions go.

Try to practice good emotions. Live courageously instead of angrily. Cultivate inner peace. Choose positively and release your anger. Live calmly and try to help God build a better world right here on Earth.

If there are times when you feel consumed by anger over the state of your health, repeat this affirmation: *Blessed Art Thou, King of the Uni-verse.* While repeating it, imagine yourself free of anger and any other negative feelings.

Another affirmation you might wish to repeat, one that will also help to soothe your angry feelings is: "*I am fearless. I am loving. I am secure. I am guiltless. I am hopeful. I am a child of God.*" Know in your heart that through these words you are connecting with God and working with the Holy Spirit to transmute anger into a calmer, more spiritual attitude.

Of all the tyrants in the world, our own attitudes are the fiercest warlords—the tyranny of the self over the self. Anger is a tyranny that you have established in your own heart and mind. Your crusade is to defeat and liberate yourself from the tyranny of fear.

Fear of Dying

When we are ill, one of our biggest fears is that we are going to die. When you get into that frame of mind, you are succumbing to the "I might not" tyranny of fear. This is a deadly tyranny that expresses itself in hopelessness and a submission to failure. "I might not live!" "I might not succeed in my healing." Thoughts like these rob us of our zest for life. It's a complete sellout; an escape door to avoid constructive, courageous, imaginative action. This sense of doom tends to turn our enthusiasm into boredom, our anticipation into pessimism, and our fire into ashes. Is this the path that will help you heal?

To dethrone this tyrant of hopelessness you must flow rather than resist. You do so by surrendering yourself to God. Instead of worrying about the unknown—the possible consequences of your disease—deal with each moment as it arises, and seek out every opportunity to visualize life-enhancing possibilities.

Invite joy into your life. It is as hungry as despair. It, too, is waiting to be invited into your heart and soul and be embraced. When you are joyful, despair caused by the fear of dying is defeated and humbled. The choice, of course, is always yours. Despair or joy. Which will it be?

There is a Kabbalistic affirmation that goes: "*Lo amut, ki echye.*" It means "I shall not die, but live and declare the works of the Lord." This affirmation suggests that you have a function to perform as God's partner—to tell the story of God and creation. It is an excellent affirmation, and one you should repeat over and over again when you are into that "I might not make it" way of thinking.

The following exercise is a very beautiful, healing, and calming one that reinforces the above idea. It is an especially good one to practice if you are seriously ill.

Exercise

Breathe deeply and slowly and try to relax. Next, place your hands over your head palms up. Repeat three times, *"Lo amut"*—I shall not die. Now, reach down with both arms as low as you can. Repeat this reaching down motion ten times. This is a gesture of humility. You have to be humble to enlist the universe's aid.

Each time you bend low, think of one bad habit or negative influence in your life that you want to get rid of. Your disease can be one of them. Each time you reach down toward the ground visualize one of these negative factors flowing from your fingertips into the earth. Get rid of it. Shake it off! Leave it buried in the earth.

When you have done his ten times, lift your hands above your head. Look at your fingers. The ten fingers represent the positive power of the Ten Commandments, or the Ten Emanations from the Tree of Life. Kabbalistically, the number ten also stands for new beginnings.

See each finger as representing something positive you want in your life—improved health, continued good health, an end to depression, and so on. Think of joyful things that have happened to you over the years. Visualize yourself getting all that you wish for.

While you are engaged in these positive thoughts, turn to the right in one circular motion. If you are too physically ill to do this, imagine yourself whirling in a sacred circle. Have you ever seen the Whirling Dervishes dance? These Muslim mystics dance in circles to symbolize the completeness of God.

As you turn in a circle shout out: *"I want to live, I want to live, I want to live."* Clap your hands, feel yourself entering a celebratory mood. Now stop and examine your fingers, again. Meditate on them and try to listen to what they may have to say to you.

Your fingers are unique. No one else has the same fingerprints as yours. Think of these fingerprints as a maze that leads to the truth. Follow their swirls and paths as they approach and join the palms. Now concentrate on the lines on your palms.

You don't need to know palmistry to continue. Simply rely on your feelings. What do you see? What do you hear? What do you feel? Do you see joy or beauty in your palms? Are you experiencing any sense of encouragement?

Don't give up if nothing comes through at first. This is a technique that very often requires practiced concentration. Repeat this exercise until you do succeed in hearing, seeing, or feeling something positive and uplifting.

Joy

As I've mentioned before, joy is an excellent way to free yourself from fear. It is through joy that you can transform and redirect "alien" thoughts that may be contributing to your disease into a health-enhancing love of God.

Are you joyful? Are you joyous even in the midst of your pain, illness, or other problems? Joy is an awareness of the *Shekinah*, the God/Goddess within. It opens the mind to receive the wisdom and healing we need.

Life is like a trip to Macy's department store. You can find everything you need, from the least expensive item to the most expensive. While there is everything purposeful and luxurious to be found there, some of us are satisfied with just standing outside the store and window shopping. But if you want to purchase a good life, if you want perfect health or happiness, you have to pay for it, with joy, with inner willingness to give service and your being, and to rejoice.

Even if you are seriously ill, do not succumb to melancholy or despair. Just as God created the universe He/She can create a healing. It may not take seven days, but why should you insist on such a timetable?

But for such a miracle to occur, you must cultivate the art of waiting in joy. Don't fight sadness with sadness. Joy, not tragedy, has a unifying force. Man was created in wisdom and joy.

Sure there are problems. Abraham had problems. Moses had problems. I have problems. Even as you read these words you may be feeling that your life is miserable, hopeless, negative, full of sickness.

But can you imagine the strength and power you would feel if you gave up that way of thinking right now? Instead of despairing, despite your pain and discomfort, believe that tomorrow you will climb your first rung to health and healing. Tomorrow you will be reborn again.

As long as life is in me I will feel grateful. That is a beautiful affirmation. It is one that traditional Jews around the world recite when they arise in the morning. It is called the *Modeh Ani.*

The first thing that comes to my mind when I get up is "I'm grateful to Thee, oh Lord, for life." I try to deliver this message to all who come to me ill or depressed. I tell my clients stories about the Baal Shem Tov who taught that the way to God and well-being lay in *simchah,* joyfulness.

So choose life! Choose joy! Always try to keep your emotions in balance—even if something uncomfortable is happening to you—and you will be well on the road to maintaining and improving your health.

There is a difference between happiness and joy. It's not a dictionary difference, but a spiritual one. Happiness is outwardly directed. You can buy happiness at Macy's or some other department store. Happiness is related to things—like a car, a beautiful home, a position, money in the bank, family, and children, but in life certain things cannot be bought for money, or material possessions. And this is where most of us make our mistake. Somehow, we feel that "If only I had money," or "if only I was married," or "if only I had children," then I would be happy.

I believe this way of thinking is the cause of many sicknesses of the heart and diseases of the soul.

Joy, on the other hand, is centered within. It is a place where you don't need things. Joy is the knowledge that we are in some way adding to the Kingdom of God, whether it's through the study of the Bible, Torah, the Kabbalah or other spiritual texts.

Do you want joy? Then be joyous. Do you want health? Then strive to be healthy. Do you want love? Then love. If you choose for your life to be joyous, to be healthy, to be worthwhile, to be meaningful and purposeful, then nothing in the world—even God—can interfere with it.

Enthusiasm

Enthusiasm is a part of joy and can dethrone fear. Enthusiasm, called *hitlahava* in the Hassidic tradition, is a necessary tool for expressing joy, experiencing awe, and allowing your spirit to cleave to God.

Cleaving to the Lord, or *devekut,* means becoming consciously certain of your oneness with the Absolute. This certainty requires *kavanah,* a form of single-minded and enthusiastic awareness of such unity.

Devekut, or cleaving, is one of the simplest and, at the same time, most complex concepts in the Jewish mystical tradition, and is very important for healing. To become one with God means simply to be at peace within, a peace that can be achieved through practices such as meditation. In meditation and other inward-directed practices we become quiet and listen to what God wants us to do.

Once you reach this state of *devekut* through meditation, you will see yourself as nothing more than a receptacle for universal truths. You will see God reflected in the clear mirror of your own soul.

Such a feeling of union with God will help you develop love, a power that is so enormous that it will literally draw the Divine into your body where it can be directed to those places that require healing.

The trick to all of this is developing *hozeh,* which means "vision," or, more specifically, holding on to that vision of seeing God in front of us all the time. Lord Krishna told his followers, "Think of me always." That is an example of *hozeh.*

And how exactly do you keep that vision of the Lord before you? There are many ways, most of them quite simple. For example, I find great pleasure in taking a walk and contemplating how trees and flowers grow.

As I walk I reflect to myself, "How wondrous are Your works, God." You can also hold a newborn baby in your arms, or watch a sunrise—almost anything from the simple to the sublime that evokes a sense of awe in you.

Moses obtained his perfect *devekut* while in a high place called Mount Sinai. Was it really a mountain or, as Kabbalistic tradition suggests, a perfect state of meditation?

During each day of our lives there are many moments when we experience a sense of awe and know that God is right in front of us. Try to increase your awareness of those special moments.

Feel the love—*ahava,* in Hebrew—and the peace that encompasses you when you are in a state of awe. Being awake to such moments will take you far along your road to better health.

To cleave to God, to experience awe, requires a great amount of enthusiasm. Without such enthusiasm, your motivation to get well may grow weak.

Lack of enthusiasm will affect your work with the Tree of Life. It will also prevent you from attaining *devekut*, which not only requires enthusiasm, but fearlessness as well.

So to dethrone fear, practice good emotions such as joy and enthusiasm, and temper those emotions, which are destructive, such as anger and melancholy. Release worries, hate, and jealousy—the prodigies of fear. Instead, choose positively and say "yes" to life. Serve the God of joy, not the God of despair.

There are two additional Kabbalistic exercises designed to dethrone fear and eliminate worry from your life. I prefer to do these exercises early in the morning after saying my morning prayers. But they may also be done at night just before you retire.

Correct Breathing

Before we get started, however, I want to introduce to you a Kabbalistic technique for proper breathing. Concentrating on the breath is important before doing any kind of metaphysical work.

The Hebrew word for breathing is *ruach*, which can also mean spirit. Breathing is taking in God's energy. When you stop breathing you stop living, so it's important to practice correct breathing.

In both the Buddhist and Hindu traditions, there are many yogic breathing exercises. The difference between breathing as taught in yoga practice and the Kabbalistic way of breath is that in the latter case when we breathe the air through our nostrils we're thinking about the *yetzer hatov*—the good inclination or our positive impulse.

When we exhale the breath from our nostrils, it is the *yetzer harah*—the negative inclination or impulse—that we focus upon. And in the intervals between each breath, we think about how God breathed life and placed His/Her spirit into the bodies of Adam and Eve.

During that moment of holding our breath we become Adam and Eve when God has infused us with his holy spirit.

According to Kabbalah, this type of concentration upon the breath was practiced by King Solomon. This great Jewish King and son of King David believed that the breath was holy and contained within it the elements of air, fire, and water. King Solomon also believed that one of the most effective ways of feeling God's presence was through the vehicle of breath. So when you do this breathing exercise, think of your breath as a channel between yourself and the Divine.

Breathing Exercise

First make a circle with the thumb and forefinger on your right hand. Then, with the remaining three fingers, close the left nostril. Now breathe in the good inclination through the right nostril.

Hold your breath for a moment or two and think positive thoughts. You may want to visualize being Adam or Eve and watch God impart His/Her healing and joyous spirit to you, or think of yourself as absolutely healthy.

Next, let the air out of the right nostril and think of the negative inclination. Concentrate on what you want to get rid of in your life—ill health, negative feelings, sadness, and so on.

Repeat the above steps, but this time close the right nostril with the last three fingers of the right hand. Repeat this exercise ten times. When you finish, repeat this affirmation. "*All is in divine order with the help of God.*"

After completing this breathing technique, you are now ready to move on to the first exercise.

Exercise 1: Find a place where you will be comfortable and not be disturbed for about fifteen minutes. Close your eyes and visualize you and God walking along a beautiful sandy beach. It can be some place you've been before or a beach that you create in your imagination.

Be aware of the fact that you are not walking "after God," as Noah is described as doing in the Bible, nor are you are walking "before God" as the Bible describes Abraham as doing. Instead, you are walking side by side with God. You and God are together, the two of you are one. Take a nice long walk with God. Remember the words of the Psalmists who said, "if you walk with God you will have no fear."

As you walk with God tell Him/Her what you want. This is the perfect moment to ask the Lord to remove fear from your life so that you can get on with your healing work. Now imagine a feeling of calmness sweeping over you.

You have released your worries, fear, and anger. You have surrendered difficulty and replaced it with God's power. Bask in this feeling of inner peace. You are no longer afraid.

Exercise 2: This Kabbalistic exercise is called "The Middle Pillar" meditation. It is based on a visualization of the Tree of Life. Find a place where you will be comfortable and away from ringing phones and other disturbances.

Close your eyes. Imagine that standing on your right side is the Archangel Michael, who is the angel of protection and balance. Michael is dressed in a flowing gold robe. On your left side stands the Archangel Gabriel, who is the angel of hope, illumination, and love. Gabriel is clothed in a red robe.

Before you stands the Archangel Ariel, who leads you to God and is the angel of vision. His robe is a dazzling combination of gold and silver. Behind you is the Archangel Rafael, the healing angel, wearing a green and purple robe. Above you is the *Shekinah*, filling you with the brilliant light of God's love.

Visualize these angels and all your fear will vanish. You are totally protected. You are not alone. What can you fear when you're surrounded by such a heavenly host whose mission is to fill us with life and energy? Stay in this meditative state until you are ready to bid the angels goodbye.

Two Divinely Powerful Ladies

"Her face shines with a light from beyond.
She basks in the oneness of the holy light."
—Zohar—

The Shekinah

According to Jewish mystical tradition, God is both masculine and feminine. Kabbalists believe that the Godhead, or the Supreme Being, is a union of male and female, and it was this union that resulted in the creation of the universe.

The *Shekinah* represents the female manifestation of deity. She, along with the *Neshama*, or soul, through the power of faith and imagination, can be enlisted to help you on your healing quest.

There is a legend that explains how the *Shekinah* entered into our lives. In the Garden of Eden Adam and Eve, God's children, disobeyed the Creator's only commandment: "Do not eat of the tree of knowledge of good and evil." One part of the Divine (the masculine part) insisted on punishing Adam and Eve. The *Shekinah*, the feminine manifestation of the Divine, did not want to punish them. "God, you can't do this. These are little children," the *Shekinah* argued. "They weren't rebelling, they just didn't know any better."

But the masculine aspect of God was unswerving. "No! If they don't learn now they will never learn. They have to go," He declared. Well, the *Shekinah* insisted just as firmly that the punishment was too great for the deed.

Finally, after arguing all afternoon, the *Shekinah* said: "If they go, I go."

So *Shekinah* went into exile away from her Bridegroom. She left with Adam and Eve and became a part of each one of us. The word *Shekinah* comes from the Hebrew word "*Shokain*," which means the one who dwells within every human being.

The story continues that after God expelled his creations—which were part of Himself as well—the Lord became very lonely. The Almighty realized that not only was He/She without any children, but also without a bride. And ever since that day The Lord has been waiting for *Shekinah* and God's children to come back home.

Although God is still waiting for the return of *Shekinah*, you need not do so. She is already there within you, along with her sister—another elegant but quiet lady—the *Neshama*, or soul.

Stay aware of and awake to the presence of the *Shekinah* and the *Neshama*, the soul. Speak to them during your meditation. Ask them if there is any way they can help you to transmute sickness into health, sadness into joy, darkness into light. Everything is possible when you are in such God consciousness. But it is up to you to make it happen.

The following meditation will help you remain aware of *Shekinah*. This meditation is best done during the evening hours. You may wish to light some white candles before you begin. Also keep pen and paper handy.

Exercise

Choose a quiet place where you won't be disturbed. For this exercise, wear only clean clothes and, if possible, wear only white. This color is helpful in leading the heart toward the love of God. Now take some calming breaths and close your eyes. Imagine that your body is being cleansed with a spiritual light.

Concentrate on the Hebrew letters that comprise God's name—*Yod, Hay, Vav, Hay*—which spell the word *Yehovah*. You may wish to write these letters down. Fill your heart with gladness and joy, because you are now in touch with *Shekinah*.

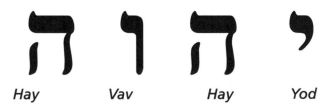

Hay   Vav   Hay   Yod

Figure 4

Whether you visualize these letters in your mind or write them down, remain mindful of them. What is it about these letters that inspires you? What new concepts and ideas do you understand that you did not grasp before?

As new thoughts and ideas fill your mind, turn all your attention to God. You are the envoy of the King, the Lord's ambassador. Ask the Maker for guidance, whether it be for your health problem or whatever else you are concerned about.

Write down whatever answers you may receive. These are God's words to you. Rejoice in the knowledge that God loves you. When your meditation on the *Shekinah* is completed, repeat the following affirmation: *Ki Tov*, it is good.

Lesson of the Candle

One day I lit a candle, and I heard the candle speak. She said to me, "Look, I'm a candle and I know what I have to do.

"Now that you lit me, I brought light into your home. And when I get down to my bottom, I will be gone. Do you know what you are supposed to do, and who you are?"

This was a lesson to me about awareness, about staying open to such concepts as the *Shekinah* and the *Neshama*. This awareness of the God and Goddesses within is important because it can help you to eliminate fear.

As I've already explained, fear and anxiety are foreign elements that don't belong in our lives. They are detrimental to wholeness and sound health. The heroic people who survived the Holocaust—people like psychoanalyst Viktor Frankl—managed to put aside their fear. They would say to themselves, "This, too, shall pass." They replaced fear with hope. If you have no hope then you have nothing.

Hope is our potential, not our present condition. You don't have to be an optimist or a pessimist if you are not feeling well, but always be a "possibilist." Encourage rebellion against fear and despair.

Cultivate the art of waiting in joy for things to change. They will if you believe they will. The power is within you. As the Baal Shem Tov once said, "You are the captain of your soul, the master of your fate."

Exercise

Light your own candle and think about it. See how it illuminates the darkness. Visualize the darkness of ill health disappearing.

Now begin to talk with the *Shekinah* and your soul. Insist on a healing. Use the combined powers of these female divinities for greater life and healing. Remember that God manifests in everyone and longs to be spoken to.

When you end this meditation, continue to create light in your life—not just with words and thoughts, but also with actions.

The Soul

"The light of the Lord is the soul of man," says Baal Shem Tov. The ancient mystics taught that the soul of man is divided into three parts. When man is born, he gets only an inferior degree of soul involvement. This is called *nefesh*.

By virtue of learning and overcoming negative inclinations, he or she may regain the next higher degree of his soul, the *ruach*. Finally, if a person has spiritually evolved, he or she reunites with the highest level of the soul, the *Neshama*. This is the closest link with God.

In the *Zohar*, the Kabbalistic "Book of Splendour," the soul is described as one of the Divine Sparks of the Supreme Being that was broken off to form the core of each living human being. These sparks were scattered during creation, and reside in everything that exists.

The power of the soul has intrigued great minds throughout history, as they sought to define its essence and release its magic. Great thinkers from Plato and Seneca to the Baal Shem Tov pondered the soul to find evidence for the existence of God, and for everything else from the soul's mission after death to its use for healing.

The soul can help change your relationship from the fear of God to the love of God. Soul power means to change your relationship from "Who am I?" to "How am I?" "How can I best manifest the God in me for health and healing?" Soul power means awareness of the divinity of man.

I first learned about "Soul Power" from the writings of the Baal Shem Tov. The founder of the Hassidic Movement was a revolutionary who was dissatisfied with the status quo and fought the rabbinical establishment. He and his disciples sought the soul in man, and through man a more reasonable, a more just, and a more loving society—a society with a soul. Out of his activities came the new concept of the *Shekinah*—the concept of the loving, caring, compassionate, and personal Living God.

According to Kabbalistic tradition, the *Neshama*, or soul, leaves the body during the night. It goes up to heaven to give a report of the daily activities. There is a night court in session, which listens to the soul.

Some souls remain there. They don't get permission to return. And the next day we find out that person has died. When I get up in the morning and I open my eyes and see my family and the sunshine I rejoice. I immediately put myself in this joyous mood because I made it! My soul has returned. How wonderful! And in gratitude, I recite the *Modeh Ani* prayer: "*I am grateful to You, living, enduring King, for restoring my soul to me in compassion....*"

A Quiet Lady

The soul is a quiet lady. She is always there but doesn't really do anything. But although she is quiet, it doesn't mean that she is not always communicating with you. The secret is to learn to listen in order to hear her.

One time my soul spoke to me quite forcefully, letting me know that I was out of balance. I was the rabbi of a congregation in Princeton, New Jersey. I was quite happy and comfortable in that quaint college town. I had a beautiful house and a very comfortable salary. After my third year there I heard my soul cry.

I ignored her the first or second time that happened. I also started getting sick more than I usually did. The third time I finally sat down and decided to meditate to find out what was bothering me inside.

I listened and what I heard was my soul telling me, "You're doing fine, you're a great rabbi, and people love you. But you're not growing. You're doing nothing for yourself.

"You have a nice home, you're comfortable, you eat well, you're doing the right thing, you preach, the body is well taken care of, but you're still not feeding the soul."

My soul told me that instead of going up the spiritual ladder, I was climbing the same rungs over and over again. In fact, she pointed out that I was actually beginning to slip downward on a couple of the rungs.

Despite everything I thought I was doing right, I was essentially leading a meaningless life. I was, she said, "not in balance."

And that's when I decided to leave my position. I wasn't leaving the rabbinate, I was leaving my attachment to that congregation. I thought, if I am so comfortably employed, how can I really be a spiritual leader? Without realizing it, I was listening more to what the board of directors was saying than my own heart.

So I left and became a "listening rabbi." Instead of preaching, instead of worrying about the board of directors and my salary, I decided to listen to what people needed and wanted and try to respond to it.

I dedicated the next forty years of my life to this kind of ministry. I eventually created my own synagogue. There was no board of directors. There was no budget. There was no salary. I had something better than all that. I had a loving and open place to worship God. One that welcomed anyone who wanted to come whether they were Christian, Hindu, Jew, or Muslim.

I still operate my "New Synagogue" in New York City this way. And I believe I have been in perfect balance since making that decision. And, thank God, at age eighty-eight, I am rarely sick.

The Soul Connection

Although the language of the soul is silence, it doesn't mean that she isn't always communicating with us. We have to learn how to speak her language, and we can do that through meditation.

When we speak about balance in a person, we always speak about keeping the body, mind, and soul in harmony. The body and the mind tell you what they need. But I believe that we have to pay special attention to the soul because the nature of the soul is quietude. We must stop being so occupied with our bodies or our minds and pay more attention to this spiritual lady. Because if she is in any way harmed, the damage can result in poor physical health.

Once you determine or suspect that your soul may be out of balance, then you've got to get right to work to correct those imbalances. One way to restore balance is through Tree of Life pathwork and meditation.

We get out of balance whenever we do things that are an affront to God. Then we're ignoring and rejecting the soul and upsetting her balance. If you remain aware of the presence of your soul, then there is less of a tendency to do the wrong thing.

Thinking about the *Neshama* serves as a reminder not to follow your evil impulses and, then the soul suffers no damage. Also, whenever you think about the soul, you know that you are more than the body, the flesh, and whatever else makes up our physical existence. The soul reminds us that there exists a spiritual dimension and that healing work can be done on this level.

The soul doesn't control your body, but it is there to help you. There was a great rabbi who was once asked, "Where is God?" And his fellow rabbi replied, "Wherever He is invited."

If you don't invite God in, you don't get any benefits. By remaining aware of the soul, you are inviting God in. The benefits, of course, are increased opportunities for spiritual healing.

If you can hear, feel, or experience the *Shekinah* and the *Neshuma* in any manner, then you have started on the road to total healing. You are bringing God into your life. You are becoming a holy missionary of the Creator, helping to change illness into health.

Your "missionary work" can lead you to become a physician of the soul—your own soul. There is no guru in the universe who can save your soul except yourself in partnership with God. Spiritual doctors like myself can certainly point you in the right direction, but the major part of this missionary work is up to you.

The following exercise that will help you get in closer touch with your soul:

Exercise

Find a quiet place where you will not be disturbed. Relax, do some breathing exercises, and think about the Hebrew word for soul, which is "*Neshama*." The ancient mystics would often describe the soul as the "light of the body."

Thinking about light immediately begins to dispel the darkness. Meditate on the fact that you have been sitting in the darkness for much to long. Confront your "heart of darkness." To get well, you want to turn things over to higher love and wisdom.

See yourself seated in a dark room. There is a switch on the wall next to you. Reach for the switch and turn it on. Now you are bathed in the light.

You now see yourself in a different way. In the light your body looks healthier. See yourself radiating health You can even see the soul glowing within you.

The *Neshama* is delighted that you have thought about her. Do you sense her joy? The healing light grows brighter. Someone else now enters the room.

It is the *Shekinah*. She nods happily, pleased at sharing the light with her sister, your soul. Spend some time discussing your problem with these two divinely powerful ladies. Ask for their guidance. Then listen carefully to the wisdom that they offer you.

Getting on the Right Road

"All depends upon his deeds."
—Zohar—

What is sickness? Sickness is a sign that something is wrong with you, and I don't mean solely in a medical sense. I'm not talking about your symptoms.

I know that there are all kinds of scientific theories about the causes of illness. There are germ theories and virus theories and theories that stress lack of oxygen. Even not drinking enough water can lead to disease.

Well, I'm a physician of the soul, not a medical doctor. So I look at things a little differently. I believe that when something goes wrong with the body, it is very often—but not always—your own creation.

When I get sick I know that I've done something wrong on some level. It may have to do with the body, or physical level—the way I eat, what I eat, not getting enough fresh air or exercise. When I talk about the importance of proper diet and exercise, I'm not speaking about sometimes having an occasional bag of M&Ms or missing a day or a month at the gym or the pool. That won't necessarily make you ill. But chronic physical, mental, emotional, and spiritual bad habits may lead to a visit to the doctor's office. The root cause of my illness may be connected with my mind. I was judgmental, filled with anger, perhaps even unforgiving of people in my life. The cause of my sickness could also have been on the spiritual or soul level. I neglected my spiritual life and that upset my soul, prompting some kind of physical reaction.

The bottom line is that I somehow became out of balance and this may have resulted in my present ailment. If you suspect that your disease may be the result of disharmony, then there are ways to return to wholeness, but you have to take the responsibility and get on the right road to reverse the situation.

Of course there are times when imbalance or disharmony may have nothing at all to do with your physical or emotional condition. There are obviously many other reasons why one becomes ill—from inherited genetic weaknesses to the poisoning of the environment. These are things over which we have little or no control. If that is your situation, then what you are experiencing is a tragedy—not a problem. And tragedies are simply something that we have to learn how to accept and live with. As bad as they may be, it does not mean you should give up on life.

I once read about a friend of the philosopher Martin Buber. This man, whose name I cannot remember, was totally paralyzed from the neck down. But he had movement in one toe. Did he give up on life? Absolutely not! This brilliant man somehow learned how to use that toe to type. He actually wrote several books using this method. I recall that in the interview he said, "Yes, I'm paralyzed, but I'm also something else. I'm an author." That is how he courageously faced the tragedy that befell him.

Tragedies aside, quite often we do develop health problems because we are out of balance on an inner level. We fail to eat properly, drink or smoke too much, ignore exercise, or slip into negative mental attitudes rather than positive ones. All of these can result in disease.

The ancient Kabbalists expressed this notion by saying, "Each time you do something good, you create an angel. And each time you do something wrong, you also create an angel—a fallen one."

I like to use the more modern metaphor of a car moving down a highway to explain illness rather than "fallen angels." Instead of concentrating on the road—symbolizing health—your thoughts drift off. Suddenly, you find that you've made a wrong turn and have gotten lost.

So you pull over and say, "I don't know where I am." Some drivers immediately do the wrong thing and continue to drive another ten or twenty miles. What kind of fallen angel are they creating? Probably an angry or frustrated one.

Other motorists who are lost will stop and ask someone for assistance. Asking for help when you are ill is a better idea. But I think the best approach is to look at your cosmic roadmap—the Tree of Life—and try to find out not only where you made the wrong turn, but why.

Certainly when you are sick it is important to seek professional help. But it is equally important to try and figure out where and why you got off the road to good health. Where did you make the wrong turn?

Some readers of this book may believe that they are on the right road because they currently have no physical symptoms. The lack of symptoms, however, is far from any accurate barometer of your physical, emotional, or spiritual state of health.

In truth, there are three kinds of people who need healing: the neurotic who always fears becoming ill, the person who is truly sick, and, yes, the normal person who says he or she is feeling perfectly fine.

But why the normal person? Because they often think that they have everything going for them. What they may not be aware of is their lack of joy or other negative emotions, which will eventually lead to poor health.

A story can illustrate this type of personality. One day I received a telephone call from a man who said he had attended my last lecture, in New York City at Carnegie Hall. He asked if he could make an appointment to see me. This man was quite wealthy, and he flew to New York all the way from Virginia.

When he sat down in my office I saw that he was very dignified, very expensively dressed, tall, and good-looking. He was a graduate of Princeton University, a very impressive man who appeared to be in the prime of his life.

We sat in silence for about two or three minutes as I waited for him to speak. Finally, he said, "You've got something." I said, "What?" He said, "You have joy." He had everything going for him but joy. This was a "normal" but not really healthy person.

Certainly there was nothing physically wrong with him. But he was spiritually empty and on some deep level sensed that his life needed an adjustment if he was to retain his health. So he commuted back and forth to my office where I began a series of healing sessions with him, which were to dramatically improve his quality of life.

This is an excellent example of a man who decided he needed to get on the right road. I wonder how many other people, whether sick or well, are aware enough to arrive at the same conclusion?

So if you have made a wrong turn, exactly how do you get back on the highway to health? The answer is through awareness. You must first have the courage to examine your life and determine whether or not your body, mind, and soul are really in balance.

You must examine your motives, your attitudes, your thoughts, and your actions. One of the best ways to do this is through a process, which I like to call the "psycho/spiritual checkup."

Psycho/Spiritual Checkup

Periodically checking your own spiritual pulse is as important as going for an annual physical. It will help determine whether or not you are living in balanced harmony.

A regular spiritual "checkup" will also help you along the path of right thinking. It will remind you that spiritual fitness requires the same kind of persistence that you devote to your physical exercise program.

You need discipline, repetition, patience, and tenacity to keep at it. Like physical exercise, you certainly cannot expect to derive benefits in only one session. And like your physical fitness program, you must keep at it even when you are feeling lazy about doing so.

Checking the level of your spiritual fitness is important because you simply can't climb the ladder to heaven if you are not ready. If you're not fit spiritually you don't belong there yet.

One way to check your spiritual fitness is to ask yourself questions like: Am I spiritually whole? Do I accept the fact that my Father/Mother and I are One? Am I aware that I am in partnership with God and that the Almighty needs me as much as I need Him/Her?

During this checkup, ask yourself whether you are striving to achieve a mature interest in other people, and throwing the bridge of love across the abyss of frustration? Ask yourself whether you believe that you can turn from monologue toward dialogue and from aloneness toward communion.

One way to check your psychological fitness is by asking yourself if you are different today than you were yesterday. This question helps to promote awareness, which always leads to good health.

Each day I look at my wife, my children, and my students. If I see them the same way that I did yesterday, then I am not growing psychologically, and something needs to be done. I am not psychologically fit.

But if even a tiny bit about them seems a little different than yesterday, then I'm on the right road. I'm growing. This is one of the important things about psychotherapy. It helps you to grow by seeing life differently each day.

So during this psycho/spiritual checkup, concentrate on what your self-image is. Who are you? Why are you? What are you? What are you to yourself? What is your connection to God? These are all meaningful questions that will help bring you into a state of self-awareness.

Once you review the results of your "checkup" and find that you are out of "shape," the most important question you must ask yourself is whether you have the courage to change your internal environment.

Take charge of your kingdom—your body—and do what you must to love God, live life with joy, focus your mind through study, be humble before God and your fellow human beings, and avoid pride, anger, frivolity, and fear.

Learn to respect the sacredness of your body and soul, and become aware that body, mind, and soul are holy places that need to be maintained and not ignored.

Once you have developed that kind of awareness, then you are ready to begin transformational healing work. So now let's get ready to replace disharmony with balance. Let's gain some self-control. As the Beatles' song goes—let us "come together" in body, mind, and soul.

Purifying Body, Mind, and Soul

"Cleanse your body and sharpen your mind."
—Kabbalistic aphorism—

In order to do any type of healing work—whether on yourself or for others—and to receive guidance from God, you have to be in a state of readiness, or *hahanah* in Hebrew. Without this state of readiness, the mystics believed you will miss the essence of things.

The ancient Kabbalists explained the importance of readiness by utilizing the metaphor of "two rooms in a house." Illness was represented by one of those rooms. Health and God's healing presence were symbolized by the second room.

The person seated in the first room has to decide if he or she is *really* prepared to enter the second room. To determine their preparedness, they are required to look at themselves in a large mirror and ask themselves this question: "Am I ready?"

What would your answer be? I know that you'd probably say yes, but think about it. Are you *really* ready for life? Have you fasted or done other purification work in anticipation of receiving God's healing hand?

How is your meditation practice? Are you feeling close to God? Are you experiencing the awe of entering the other room? Are you psychologically prepared so that your ego, fear, or skepticism will not interfere with your faith?

Have you diligently been trying to replace melancholy and pessimism with a spirit of hope and enthusiasm? What were the results on your last psycho/spiritual checkup? This is all part of the process of *hahanah* before you can enter the next room.

Sometimes I will suggest to my Kabbalah students that they should read a certain book. By the next class some students tell me that they have already finished reading it. Then I ask them, "What did you learn?"

Most of these speed readers will say, "I don't remember," and yet they want to get on with the rest of their lessons. They're in a hurry, but they're not even ready to discuss the book they've just read.

Read a book slowly, sentence by sentence. If it's a book about health, make sure you're absorbing it. After one or two sentences you should close your eyes and see the words in your mind's eye. For healing work, you must get ready in the same slow and deliberate manner.

Some of my clients tell me they are ready for healing because they know all the right affirmations, all the proper meditations. They tell me they've done reiki, and shiatsu, and yoga.

I tell them that all of that is wonderful, and ask them if they are ready to experience the moment when they open the door to the next room. Is their body clean, their mind pure, and their soul cleansed of negative thoughts?

If not, then they are not in a state of *hahanah*. We must do things in the proper order to expect healing from God. Preparing yourself for *hahanah* is no light task. In truth, this type of preparation never ends.

The first step in getting ready is a purification ritual. Before Native American medicine men begin any healing work, they enter a sweat lodge to purify themselves. In Judaism we have our own version of the sweat lodge. It is called the *mikvah*, or ritual bath. Orthodox Jewish women usually do this purification ritual once a month. According to Hassidic tradition, men—especially students of Kabbalah—purify themselves in the *mikvah* each day.

There's no need to buy yourself a new bathing suit. Instead, I will teach you a simple technique that symbolizes our immersion in the waters of purification—the Jewish version of baptism. Once we finish purifying the body, then we will purify the mind and spirit as well.

Purifying the Body

Historically, a person immersed themselves in the hot water of the *mikvah* three times. The first immersion represented death. The second one signified burial, and the third immersion is symbolic of renewal. You are born, again.

The essential purpose of the *mikvah* is not to cleanse the body—you're not taking a bath—but to purify and make holy the temple, which contains mind and soul.

In the Hindu tradition, as well as many others, such a purification ritual is essential. One Vedic pearl of wisdom commands: "Keep the mind pure, the body clean, the life well-disciplined, the heart dedicated, and this is yoga."

Since ritual baths are a bit hard to find nowadays unless you live in an orthodox Jewish community, for our purposes we are going to create a symbolic *mikvah*, using only our hands. We build our *mikvah* with our ten fingers.

The ten fingers represent the ten spheres or *sefiroth*—the ten attributes of Divinity—that comprise the Tree of Life. These attributes are Divinity, Wisdom, Knowledge, Compassion, Judgment, Beauty, Victory, Glory, Foundation, and the Kingdom. I will discuss the spheres of the Tree of Life later in this book.

The fingers also represent the Ten Commandments. In addition, ten is a mystical Kabbalistic number that symbolizes new beginnings, which is especially auspicious for those of us who are seeking to transform illness into good health.

Exercise

Take a small bowl and fill it with hot water. Dip your ten fingers in the water three times. Close your eyes for a moment and feel the purifying heat of the water going through your whole body.

Repeat the Hebrew word "*tahor*," which means "I am clean, sanctified, purified." Then dry your fingers carefully and put your hands together palm to palm and fingertip to fingertip.

This action symbolizes the positive aspect of our personality—the right hand—and the negative inclination—the left hand—merging to recreate the idea that All is One.

You are now seated in the *mikvah* of your mind. God's healing light streams through a window. It is warm and healing. Think about this concept for a few minutes and let the purifying light of the spirit of God wash over you and cleanse your body.

Breathe in this light and then breathe it out. These are the breaths that Adam took, which gave him life. You are now breathing in new life. Kabbalistically, this light is known as *ruach Elohim*, the spirit of God. Feel it coursing throughout your body and healing any areas that are giving you discomfort.

Purifying the Mind

To purify the mind so that it may receive divine guidance for healing work, we, again, use the analogy of light. The mind symbolizes light, as you can readily see when two people are arguing and one says, "Ah, yes, now I *see* what you mean." When we understand, it's like a light going on.

Kabbalists traditionally light two candles. This is also done in Jewish homes on Friday night to celebrate the Sabbath, and on many holidays as well.

Lighting two candles symbolizes that each of us is comprised of the *Yetzer hatov*, the so-called good inclinations, and the *Yetzer harah*, the so-called bad inclinations.

There is a constant war going on between these two impulses. By combining these two candles, we are now creating harmony. We are joining the positive and negative until they become one great torch of light so that you no longer know which is which. All you do know is that the darkness has disappeared, and now there is light.

There are a variety of other ways to purify and prepare the mind for healing work. One suggestion is to read spiritual literature such as the Bible. Meditation is another effective method.

If you choose to meditate, focus on clearing your mind of any thoughts of fear, anxiety, hatred, or anything negative. Try to replace such thoughts with images that reflect more spiritual awareness.

The following exercise can help you purify your mind. It is called the "Let There Be Light" meditation.

Exercise

Find a comfortable place where you will not be disturbed. Relax by doing some breathing exercises. Next, close your eyes and visualize the two candles, which symbolize both sides of your personality, the positive inclinations and the negative inclinations.

Feel the harmony of the two flames becoming one. Repeat the words, "*Ki tov, ki tov,*" it is good!" Feel yourself establishing a real communication with God.

You are now speaking to the Lord. You are telling God that you love Him/Her and the Creator is returning that message of love. According to Kabbalistic tradition, through this two-way communication you are now creating the upper world and the lower world, which are actually both one.

Now repeat to yourself the following affirmation: *I am happy. I am healthy. I am satisfied. I am glad to be alive.* Feel the excitement and the joy of living.

When you feel this strong link between the two worlds, you have attained a mystical state which the Kabbalists call *hitlahavuth*—the fervor, the excitement, the joy of living. You are now prepared to receive God's healing energy.

Purifying the Soul

Now that your body and mind have been purified, let's turn our attention to the *Neshama*, or soul. It is not always easy to figure out exactly how to purify one's soul.

There is a Hassidic story that serves to illustrate the problem. Two rabbis were preaching all over the country. One was more learned than the other. By chance, the two of them met in a little village. The less enlightened rabbi asked his peer, "Tell me, when you come to a learned community and they ask you questions to which you have no answers, what do you do?" The more learned rabbi pondered the question for a few moments and then replied: "I sing a melody."

If you are at a loss for an answer to the question, How do you purify the soul?, try singing.

That is what I do. I sing a beautiful Hassidic melody to purify my soul in preparation for my healing work. The song I sing is impossible to translate from the Hebrew, but the words roughly mean, "I am ready." Ready for what? I am ready to do the good and the beautiful.

Any spiritual song can be used, including such old favorites as "He's got the whole world in His hands." If you don't like to sing, listen to a CD or tape of sacred music for a while with your eyes closed. Imagine this music washing over and purifying your soul.

Another profound way to prepare and purify the soul for healing work is to meditate on the words of the *Shemah*, the best-known Jewish prayer Shemah Yisrael. "Hear O Israel, the Lord Your God, the Lord is One."

The *Shemah* is an affirmation of faith. It both expresses our love for God, and also serves as an ode to the divinity of the soul. It brings us into a consciousness of the Oneness of God, opening our awareness that God is without and within.

The following two exercises will help you purify your soul.

Exercise

Close your eyes and make yourself comfortable. You may wish to switch off the light, so that you use only your inner light to guide you on your spiritual journey.

You are going to take a trip to the Holy Land. Somewhere on the outskirts of Jerusalem is a cave. It is a cave, according to tradition, where Jewish mystics hid to study the Torah and Kabbalah during the dark years of Roman persecution.

You are now in that cave. Sit down on the floor and exhale three times to symbolically rid yourself of all the poisons we carry around that cause disease—the poison of hate, the poison of jealousy, the poison of ignorance. Now inhale three times, symbolically taking in the blessings of being, caring, and rejoicing in one another.

Kabbalah teaches that revelation is a continuous process, and that God is ready and willing to speak to each one of us every time we are ready to listen. So while we are still in the cave, let's spend the next moments with a powerful intent to hear God's message.

Be open to different ways of hearing God speak. Listen with your spiritual "third ear" and see with your "inner eye." Feel a strong sense of awareness and dedication.

If this exercise is done properly, I am certain that the One who speaks to each one of us whenever we are ready will speak to you. Listen carefully. What you hear may be your mantra, your message in life.

When you are ready to leave the cave, repeat the mantra or message you have received. If you have not received a health-promoting mantra during your meditation, don't fret. Repeat the following meditation, which I am fond of using: *"I am ready, I am ready, I am ready. I am ready for perfect health. I am ready to accept all good and beauty."* Repeat this mantra several times. As you do, imagine a soothing feeling of peace settling over you.

If you aren't able to take the time to do the exercise described above, you can practice the following purification ritual while taking a shower in the morning. It is based on the image of the Tree of Life and is called the "Kabbalistic Shower."

Exercise

First take a bath and wash yourself thoroughly. Follow this bath with a shower to further purify yourself. While you are standing under the running water, visualize yourself being purified by divine energy.

Be fully aware of what you are doing. Allow the grace of God to flow over you and into you. Now, meditate on this affirmation: *We are the hands, the feet, and mind of God. There is peace and health and joy where we are.*

Let the water run over your head, the highest or primary generative force for God's healing. This is where the spirit of God enters your body. Next, turn to the left and let the water run down the left side of your body.

Then face forward, bring your hands together in front of you palms up, and let the water run into your hands. This helps to evoke the Archangel Michael for protection.

Next, turn to the right and let the water run down the right side of your body. Face forward again, and let the water run onto your heart, signifying beauty.

Now reach up over your head with both hands and then slowly reach down to your feet. Let the water run down your back. You are creating an endless circle, which is the symbol of God.

When you leave the shower say, "Hallelujah," or "Praise God." Spend a moment in silence and then say *"ki tov."* "Praise life!"

Moving Towards Wholeness

"The steps of a good man are ordered by the Lord."
—Psalm 37:23—

Now that you have successfully purified body, mind, and soul in preparation for your journey through the Tree of Life, the next step toward wholeness is to bring these physical, mental, and emotional energies into harmony.

The threefold path to harmony is to nourish the body, control negative feelings, and develop spiritual eyes. This will help you replace discord with harmony, and point the way to your self-chosen goal, which is wholeness and health.

Mental Health

Regardless of your present state of health, one of the most important challenges you face is to free yourself from spiritual afflictions of the mind such as hatred, guilt, anger, fear, and anxiety.

This can be quite a daunting challenge. You can start paving the way by trying not to worry about what happened yesterday or what might happen tomorrow. *Today is the day, the only day.* Worries about yesterday or tomorrow will result in tension, fear, and anxiety. This is the road toward disease.

In my experience as a trained psychotherapist I have observed that, when tension is internalized, it can "break" the heart and may even cause heart failure. Tension can put pressure on the brain and may cause a stroke. It can harden the joints and result in arthritis. Tension and anxiety can eat away at vital organs and spawn cancers and a host of other illnesses.

If it is good health that you desire, then you must learn to tame tension and anxiety. This is done by first rooting out the underlying causes, and then substituting a new way to handle life's challenges. It is called emotional maturity.

Emotional maturity means learning how to be "give oriented" and accepting rather than being "take oriented." It is when we find satisfaction in giving that we achieve a high level of emotional maturity and a reduction in tension.

Too often we act like little children wanting this and that. We feel, for example, that if only we had more money, if only we were married, if only we had a husband or wife and children. If only, if only, if only, then all would be well. We feel that we're somehow missing something and not getting enough out of life, and this can cause high levels of anxiety.

Do you remember when you were a child and were walking through a department store? Perhaps you thought, "If only I had a bike," or, "If only I had that pair of roller skates." If only, if only, if only, then I would be happy." This kind of "take oriented" attitude leads to nothing but unhappiness and can ultimately result in poor health.

Instead, be grateful for what God has given you and repay that gratitude by becoming loving and joyful. When you awaken—even if you are not feeling well—be joyful instead of *kvetching* (complaining) "if only I felt better." Love this day as the great gift from God that it is. This joyful attitude helps to eliminate tension and opens us up to the blessings of good health.

In the Jewish tradition, the purpose behind the *Bar Mitzvah* and *Bat Mitzvah* is to help create a mental atmosphere of emotional maturity. It is an ancient coming of age ritual that symbolizes giving up one's childish responses, among them, that anxious "gimme this and gimme that" or "I want this, I want that" state of mind.

Emotional health also means not giving into despair. A young man I once counseled learned this lesson well. Alfred had a life-threatening disease, and I sensed that his despair and corresponding melancholic attitude was worsening his condition.

I told this young man that despair was worse than sin, and that to give in to it was an admission of having exchanged freedom for slavery. In a state of despair one is saying that I am no longer free to utilize the

"I" in me—the "I" that Kabbalists believe is the manifestation of the spark of the divine in man.

Alfred paid attention to what I had to say and, together, we began our journey to healing. This young man had the courage to examine his motives—to explore why he had given up hope for any improvement in his medical condition.

Today, Alfred is a very active member of my congregation. Despite the predictions of his doctors, his disease remains in remission. I believe that through an adjustment in Alfred's emotional state of mind, he has found the will to live.

Alfred learned that by becoming a partner with God, miracles can happen. Once he began to believe that, this young man was able to shift his psychological emphasis from despair to hopefulness.

Should a health situation cause you to despair, take a deep breath and ask yourself during meditation, "Where do I stand?" Do I really think my situation is hopeless or is it only a fearful or anxious reaction?

Another question you might ask is, "Am I exaggerating my illness? Interestingly enough, some people take pride in this. "I am sicker than you." "I'm more tired than you." "I have been hopeless longer than you."

To such people, illness can serve as a status symbol. They love to say things like, "I've been in therapy for ten years now." This is a form of negative thinking, and the negation of life cannot make for living.

We always need to affirm life, not deny it. Affirmations are important in any kind of healing work because they set the stage for us to act positively during each day of our lives.

The Baal Shem Tov taught that the greatest sin you can commit is to despair for the future—to worry unnecessarily or become depressed. "Never permit yourself to become melancholy," he would instruct his followers.

He taught that there is but one plan to life, and that was to live life here and now. "Live in joy!" the rabbi would often exclaim. "Live in the name of God!" So if you want to move toward wholeness, then you must remain aware and try to master your negative emotions.

Too often we do not realize that we have created our own mental tyrants. We allow fear or anger to replace reason. It is vital to try and replace such negative emotions with more positive feelings. Replace these stumbling stones with stepping stones. As the eminent psychologist Fritz Perls once noted: "To suffer one's death and be reborn is not easy." But try, anyway.

Physical Health

According to the Kabbalah, in order to experience wholeness, the body needs to be cared for as much as the mind and soul. It is, after all, the physical receptacle, which contains mind and soul. Without the body, there would be no sanctuary for God to dwell in.

But this vehicle is quite vulnerable, and can be afflicted by a variety of illnesses and diseases. I believe the way we eat, how we eat, and why we eat can cause the greatest harm to the body. Proper eating is a theme that occupies much of Kabbalistic literature.

In the Bible God seems to suggest that we live a vegetarian lifestyle. In the Bible, the Creator tells us to eat the "grass of the earth." Even the Jewish word, "kosher," means to eat what benefits your body. The Biblical prohibition against eating pork and certain other types of food was also designed to protect the body from disease.

So the next time you are tempted by a cheeseburger with fries, remember that the body is the holy container of the mind and the soul and that it needs to be treated with respect. If you remain ignorant of the importance of diet and nutrition, then you are working against your own well-being.

If your body is not well, then your thinking is not right, and your actions are not right. You can have all the money in the world, but if you're in pain or discomfort, it's very difficult to function. This is why God wants us to be in good health. After all, how can we focus on prayer or worship our Maker if we are ill?

So by eating healthy—and by this I mean a mostly vegetarian diet— we can promote wholeness. It takes more energy for the body to digest food than almost anything else it does. If you are an excessive meat eater, you are not only slowing down your metabolism, but also inhibiting spirit perception.

For good health, go "eat grass" as God suggests. Other consciousness-raising foods that you should include in your diet are fish, plenty of fruits and vegetables, whole grains, nuts, seeds, and legumes. If you must eat meat, make it white meat like chicken or turkey.

I am a Kabbalistic rabbi, not a medical doctor. So the way I approach the subject of food is slightly different from that of the scientific community. To me, food always has a religious significance.

The Christian Eucharist, for example, is symbolized by drinking wine and eating a wafer. At the beginning of the Jewish New Year, the wish for a sweet year is symbolized by dipping apple slices into honey. There are many other examples of the close connection between food and spirituality. Be mindful of the food you eat and your relationship to this food. You are not only feeding your body, but, symbolically, your spirit as well. By feeding the body properly you are also nourishing the soul—the primary conductor of your state of health. I believe that a spiritual person has less of a tendency to become ill than someone who is not spiritual because a truly spiritual person doesn't overeat. A truly spiritual person has respect for their body and a certain dignity about how they treat it.

A spiritual person, in general, does not eat red meat, nor do they ingest other harmful substances such as cigarette smoke, sugar, or alcohol.

Overeating is another problem you must try to bring under control. Say you're hungry. Probably you could have satisfied your hunger with half of the food you ate. So why did you eat all of it? Because it was there. This is a gluttonous rather than a spiritual approach.

When you overburden the digestive system you are looking for trouble. How many of you eat while standing up, or rush through a meal? Where are you rushing to? Where's the fire?

My former wife was home ill for several years before she died. She couldn't eat by herself, so I would feed her. One day I was giving her a second spoonful of cereal for breakfast, and in the middle of that spoonful she was gone—she died. It took just one second. Even to this very day, I still can't get that image out of my mind. One minute she was alive and the next… So where are you rushing to? Don't you realize that in just one second we can be gone?

What you put into your body affects your future, and your future not only affects your friends and family, but your relationship to the

Almighty as well. You should not only pay attention to what you put into your body, but your state of mind while you are doing so.

Most of the time we gossip when we eat. Each time we do that we take in some poison. Little by little that poison emerges as some form of sickness. So be careful what you talk about over a meal. Better still, try not to talk at all and concentrate on the sheer joy of eating.

There's a story I like to tell about an American Jew who came to Europe to visit an old friend—a Hassidic rabbi. They hadn't seen each other for thirty years.

Over lunch, the American kept inquiring about people in the small town where the rabbi lived. "How's Rabbi Yonkel?," the American inquired. "Dead," replied the rabbi as he continued to concentrate on his noon meal. The American nodded sadly. "How's Rabbi Shlomo?" he then asked. "Dead," the Hassid said, chewing slowly on his slice of bread.

The conversation went on like this until the frustrated American exploded. "Is everybody in your town dead?" The Hassid calmly looked up from his meal. "Only when I'm eating." The moral of this story, of course, is that the rabbi refused to gossip about anyone during his meal because it would interfere with his digestion.

You don't have to be a student of Kabbalah to know that regular physical exercise, breathing exercises, restful sleep, and relaxation are all very important for the health of the body. All this takes is what we call in Yiddish *seichal*, or common sense.

A body that is fed food that honors life (the killing of animals does not), that is well rested, and that is given enough exercise is one that will respond with good health all the way down to the cellular level.

How you treat your body should not be a second-best compromise. To partake of life means to be hungry, not only hungry for freedom, or hungry for union with God, but also hungry for the right foods and physical regime that will promote vitality.

I also believe in meditative silence while dining. In our "gab-gab" culture, I know how difficult this practice can be, especially when we're having "power lunches" or entertaining friends.

Such silence can actually be an active, tender, and feeling form of communication. In monasteries around the world, meals are eaten in silence. The Zen masters say that "those who know do not speak, and those who speak do not know."

Of course, the choice is yours as to whether you wish to engage in this practice or not. But you should at least be aware that digestion is vastly improved when you are quietly concentrating on the taste and texture of the meal before you.

One of the greatest wrongs we commit against our body is discussing mundane matters—or even reading—while we eat. These are all distractions that separate us from the sacredness of this moment.

Although I believe meditative silence is the best way to eat one's meals, if you feel compelled to have a conversation why not focus it on some spiritual matter?

I recognize that unless you're a cleric or living in some ashram this is not likely to happen. And that's too bad. You should follow the example of most Hassids who, when they eat, discuss *Torah* over their meals. When was the last time you discussed scripture over a meal, or even discussed a subject such as the joy of life?

Another thing to keep in mind is that when food arrives at your table, you are now receiving God's blessings. He/She somehow made this food possible. At this moment it is up to you to sanctify it.

Contemplate the food that you are eating. Meditate on the One who created it. Pray over it before you eat. These are all gestures of gratitude and should be done before and after dining.

By doing so, you are also promoting harmony within yourself—a balance of mind, body, and soul. Contemplation or prayer establishes an grateful attitude and this positive frame of mind can lead to better digestion and improved health.

Spiritual Health

Life has no meaning if it doesn't include its mysteries. Life must be embraced with a curiosity for the mystical, the sublime, the unknowable. This is what spirituality is all about.

Spirituality enlarges the personality. It expands our vision. Everything —including improved health—is possible when you are in God consciousness, no matter how you may be feeling.

I am always trying to develop my spiritual eyes. One way I do so is by taking a walk in the morning. The walk often leads me to a bridge. I stand under the bridge and I see all the trucks delivering goods to the city. I stand in awe. I think about all the energy, the work that went into the products that these trucks are delivering.

By the way, I believe awe is the greatest component of spirituality. This feeling of awe helps to keep you in God consciousness. Awe is not only good preventive medicine, but also an excellent healing tool.

It is through a sense of awe that we negate the frightened solitude of the Existentialists—a solitude that can lead to many debilitating effects. When we experience awe of our Creator, our soul unfolds itself like a "lotus of countless petals" and helps the physical body to bloom.

Perhaps the most effective way to improve your spiritual health is by opening yourself to more love. There is no commandment in the Bible to eat, drink, or sleep. However, there is a commandment to love. Because love is not always simple to accomplish, we are commanded to love. The implication is that this is a commandment we must work on.

Why must you love? There are many reasons, but let me offer you a very simple one. It will make you feel better on a psychological, physical, and spiritual level. Love power generates a chain reaction which brings you closer to God. And the closer you get to God the better you will feel. You will develop this "I belong to God, and God belongs to me" state of mind. What an impetus for healing!

So to open your spiritual eyes you must practice love, not only towards God, but to yourself and your fellow man as well. Such a loving attitude will not only bring you personal joy, but freedom from repressed hostility, guilt, and anxiety—negative feelings that can create emotional and physical problems.

Your spiritual health can also be harmonized by entering the "secret place of the most high" through daily meditation or through daily prayer. Try to listen to the sound of a Mighty Presence with your whole being when you meditate or pray. Become one with the expression "I am all ears" and earnestly seek spiritual guidance in your life.

The following exercise will help you to become conscious of the importance of maintaining spiritual health in order to help bring about healing. Practice this technique the next time you sit down to eat with a family member or a good friend.

Exercise

Just before you are about to eat, press your right palm to your dining companion's left palm. The combining of the right palm with the left—the positive with the negative—suggests that we are at peace with ourselves and each other.

Next, recite a prayer of thanksgiving for the food before you. Choose any prayer that you are accustomed to, or choose one from the back of this book. Think not only about God when you utter this prayer of thanksgiving, but also about the farmer who got up at 3 A.M. to work the land that produced what you are about to eat. Think of the workers who harvested the crop, the many people involved in transporting the goods to your city, and all the hands that were involved in getting your food to the supermarket shelves. Give your blessing to all the people that were involved in producing and packaging that piece of bread you are about to eat.

Healing Modalities

"I am God who heals you."
—Exodus—

Every religious tradition has its own system of healing work. All of these techniques, from the "Blessing Way" rituals of Native American medicine men to the laying on of hands of the Christian charismatics, rely on drawing power in one form or another from the universal Source of Life.

In Jewish mysticism a variety of healing techniques are employed, from the chanting of God's sacred names, to enlisting the aid of Archangels. At my Friday night Sabbath services, we perform a beautiful and very moving healing ritual in which the healing archangel, Rafael, visits our little synagogue.

When my assistant rabbi and I walk up and down the aisle in an open-eyed meditation, the Archangel Rafael works through us and offers healing to anyone in our congregation who may need it.

The use of such angelic guides are also important in my private healing work. I always feel the presence of archangels like Rafael and Michael, who is the angel of protection and balance.

There are several Kabbalistic healing modalities that intuitively open up our contact with the Divine.

Sacred Names

In Kabbalah names, like symbols, are believed to possess magical powers. There was even a ritualistic exercise that the early Kabbalists practiced called "putting on the names."

These mystics actually clothed themselves in robes that were inscribed with all the sacred names of God. This costume was an external reminder of the power that these holy names contained.

While wrapped in this mystic gown, the Kabbalist would begin an undistracted meditation on God's various holy names. This would eventually induce some kind of visionary experience, which provided answers to the mystic's questions.

The ancient Kabbalists also stressed that the invocation of God's names did not compel the Creator to respond to the will of the mystic who invoked the Divine Presence.

Even today's Kabbalists believe that they can increase their power by chanting such sacred names. They identify with the centuries of power enfolded in the use of these holy names, confident that by reciting God's names they will be connected to the all-powerful source of healing.

This sense of connection is also why prayer is so important in healing. It automatically connects you to a healing source of power. For your prayer to be effective, you must experience a deep, from the heart, connection with the Almighty when you do pray.

The following story illustrates the importance of calling upon God from the heart and soul rather than from the intellectual faculties.

There was a wealthy Jewish lady who lived along Park Avenue. This woman was well-educated and spoke French and a couple of other languages as well. She was in the hospital giving birth and was surrounded by two or three nurses.

The woman began to scream and call upon God in French. "Monsieur, monsieur, I'm suffering," she shouted. The startled nurse called the woman's doctor, Dr. Schwartz.

The doctor asked the nurse what his patient was screaming about, because he didn't understand French. When the nurse translated what she was saying, the doctor replied: "Let her scream."

Two hours later the woman was screaming again. This time she was shouting, "Jesus help me, help me." Again, the nurse called the patient's doctor. Dr. Schwartz listened and said, "Let her scream."

Several hours later the nurse was back on the phone with the doctor. "What is she screaming now?" he asked.

"Shemah Yisrael," the nurse replied. (This is the holiest prayer in the Jewish tradition.) "I'll be right over," the doctor said. He knew that this time the cry came straight from her heart—from her own spiritual tradition. The rest of her implorings were intellectual concepts that she had picked up along the way.

So if you want to draw power for your healing from the highest source, you must cry out from the heart. It doesn't matter if you're Christian, Hindu, or Muslim. What does matter is that your plea for help comes from the deepest and most authentic level of your soul.

Chanting of one of God's sacred names can also help you to remove fear from your life. You are calling upon your partner who is always there to lend a hand. You are also acknowledging your awareness of your union with spirit, and that is almost certain to light up the darkness.

Kabbalists believe that by repeating God's name, you are binding yourself to the spiritual world, and such binding opens a channel for Divine assistance. So do as the mystics do. Practice this closeness and oneness with God—called *yichud*—and it will help to bring healing energy into your life.

Exercise

Find a quiet, comfortable place where you will not be disturbed. Do some of the breathing exercises discussed earlier in this book (see chapter 3). You will be doing some enthusiastic chanting in this exercise, so find a location where you won't annoy your family or your neighbors.

Now, choose one of God's Holy Names that you most resonate with. It may be *Adonai, Adoshem, El, Yehovah, Ein Soph,* or *Rebono Shel Olam*—which translates into "Master of the Universe." You may certainly select a Holy Name from your own spiritual tradition—Jesus, Allah, Great Spirit, Buddha, or Krishna.

Chant the name you have selected seven times. Chant it with gusto and with a loving and joyful heart. However, if you are not the chanting type, it is perfectly all right to repeat the name you selected during a silent meditation while imagining the force and power behind this name.

Bring all the emotion you can muster into the repetition of this name. Do so for eight minutes. This is the Kabbalistic number which symbolizes God's name.

As you repeat the name, try to feel the presence of the *Shekinah* within. Receive the flow of divine energy. Now send that energy within you to places that may need healing.

Next, take a few deep breaths, relax, and think of yourself as healed. Imagining that result is a powerful affirmation of faith. I believe that by visualizing your prayer as one that has already been answered, you are taking action in an optimistic way.

You are affirming your faith and are preparing yourself to expect good results. From this point on simply be aware of improvements in your condition. Feel a sense of gratitude for the healing that you have been given from the Source of All Life. Say, "*Ki tov*," it is good.

Prayer

Kabbalists consider prayer to be a "courtship" between man and God. It is the simplest and most direct way to reach the Supreme Being, and an excellent method of inducing *kavanah*, the mystical cleaving to God.

All that is required when you pray is that you do so with deep feelings. Let the prayers come from your heart. Lack of enthusiasm while praying is definitely not the way to capture God's attention.

For meaningful prayer you need to be employ feelings, emotion, concentration, devotion, and directed consciousness—not the mechanical mumbling of words that we hear too often during religious services.

It is also vital that you experience a sense of joy during prayer. The prayers of the Hassids are good examples of how to pray. Enter a Hassidic synagogue on the Sabbath or on some holiday and you will find plenty of spiritual fervor.

These long-bearded men dressed in traditional black garb clap hands, sing, cry out, and sometimes even dance, as they ecstatically pour out their love and devotion to God.

Remember not to confuse prayer and meditation. Meditation turns us inward, prayer is a complete turning of the heart to the Creator. It is directed outward to the Source of All Life.

Don't be in a rush when you pray. Unfortunately, too many of us seem to be in a hurry. Maybe we have a golf game or lunch on our minds. Such distracting thoughts should not be allowed to disturb your concentration while at prayer.

So slow down when preparing to greet your Maker. Think about the scripture that proclaims, "God is in heaven and you are upon the earth. Do not rush to speak."

While it is true that God "is in heaven," it is important to understand that He/She is also within you. To really communicate with God, I think it is vital to understand and accept that concept.

At this point, you may ask what is the best prayer? To me, nothing carries more spiritual weight than the *Shemah* (see page 81). This prayer not only affirms the completeness of God, but it also suggests that God and His/Her creations are One. It is the basic and essential concept of Judaism.

What the *Shemah* tells us is that it doesn't matter what religion or race you are, because we all have the same Creator. It doesn't matter if we are young or old, male or female, sick or healthy. God is in harmony with himself and with us. You and God are One.

Meditating on the *Shemah* when you are ill will help bring you to the highest awareness of God. It will open your heart to a state of joy that can lead to healing. It will help to create harmony between your spiritual and physical selves.

When you utter this prayer, let each word "vibrate" in your mind. Feel the power of each word. Orthodox Jews repeat the *Shemah* five times each day. If you are in need of healing, you may wish to repeat this meditation five times a day.

Always concentrate on the idea that you and God are One when reciting this prayer. Remember the terms of your partnership—that both you and the Creator have a vested interest in your good health. Have faith that from this union will come new life and healing.

In the back of this book I have included several prayers used at my Kabbalistic healing center. For the following exercise you may use one of them, or choose a prayer from any spiritual tradition that suits you. Any of the holy books—from the Old Testament to the Koran—are filled with life-enhancing prayers that you may use.

This exercise, which I have done all of my life, is one of my personal favorites. It helps to set the stage for a worshipful, meditative atmosphere.

Exercise

Choose one night in the late evening to sit alone in a dark room with a single candle for illumination. The practice is especially important on Thursday night, because it gives you the opportunity to begin your mental preparation for the Sabbath that begins on the following evening.

Sit on the floor feeling humble and at one with the earth. Remember how precious every moment of your life is. Now praise God for raising you from the dust to which you shall someday return.

In your mind imagine the heavens and dwell on the mystery of creation. Repeat the *Shemah* or any prayer of your choosing. One prayer I frequently recite in addition to the *Shemah* is:

I thank you God for this healing. I let go of any fear, doubt, or negativity, which divides me from this knowledge. Blessed are you, Lord, who heals the sick. Amen.

Continue meditating on these words for as long as you like.

Psalms

These devotional poems have been used for healing in both the Judaic and Christian religions for centuries. The psalms are a cloak of many different colors. There are hymns of praise and worship, prayers for help, pleas for protection, and even requests for forgiveness.

The earliest psalms date back to the time of King David (1065–1015 B.C.), and are as enlightened in their ethics as they are lofty in their religious spirit. Offering your praise to God through the psalms connects you with more than two thousand years of spiritual history.

Praying the psalms also unites us with the unending and perfect praise and prayer of heaven and earth. You need not pray all the psalms to effect a healing. Choose one that fits your present need and circumstances.

Make a conversation and prayer out of your recital of the psalms. Yearn for God, long for God—even cry out and beg God to help you if need be. Like prayer, what is important is that the words come from your heart and that you feel love for the Lord from deep within your soul.

One of my own favorite psalms is Psalm Six, which I have adapted in the appendix to this book for your use. This psalm is both a petition for Divine help and an affirmation that such assistance is already on its way.

If you are lonely, hurting, or thirsting for a healing, another wonderful psalm is Psalm 63.

O God, you are my God,
earnestly I seek you;
my soul thirsts for you,
my body longs for you,
in a dry and weary land
where there is no water.

A psalm which can bring you much solace if you are ill, experiencing extreme stress, or worried is Psalm 63:6–8 in which David talks about his partnership with God.

On my bed I remember you;
I think of you through the watches of the night.
Because you are my help,
I sing in the shadow of your wings.
Your right hand upholds me.

Let David's psalms inspire you not to be afraid to come to God for help. Use the psalms as a way to express your true feelings and needs. Reciting the psalms will always help to lift your spirit.

Healing Touch

The hand has always played an important symbolic role in Kabbalistic rituals. The ten fingers represent the Ten Commandments and the ten *sefiroth* of the Tree of Life.

When the ancient priests performed blessings, they would separate the first three fingers from the last two fingers on each hand as they were raised in supplication. It has been suggested that this gesture symbolized the dividing of the Red Sea, proof of God's great powers.

In the old *Star Trek* television show, Spock would hold up his right hand and spread his fingers, as did the Hebrew Levite priests, when he made his greeting of peace.

Even, today, hand gestures are important. Why do we put our two hands together when we pray? The right hand represents our so-called

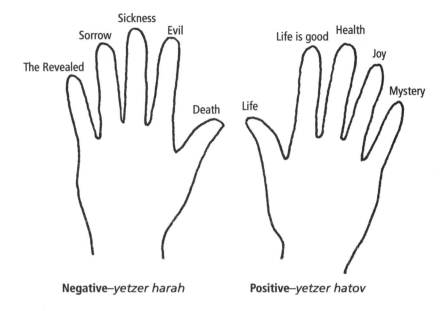

Sickness
Sorrow   Evil
The Revealed
Death   Life
Life is good   Health
Joy
Mystery

Negative–*yetzer harah*   **Positive–***yetzer hatov*

Figure 5: Hand Symbolism

positive side—the *yetzer hatov*—and the left hand represents the *yetzer harah*—our negative or evil impulses. Instead of dividing our tendencies we unite them and say to our Heavenly Father, "We are now at peace. Peace within and peace without."

According to the Kabbalah, the fingers on each hand are also symbolic.

On the right hand, the thumb symbolizes life. The forefinger represents life is good. The middle finger is the symbol for health. The ring finger represents joy, and the little finger symbolizes mystery.

Maybe that's why during the Passover service we dip our little finger into a cup of wine at one point during the *seder*. It symbolizes the mystery of that amazing event in Jewish history with all its attendant miracles—a time when God brought plagues on the Egyptians, split the Red Sea, and demonstrated other phenomena to free the Jews from bondage.

On the left hand, the thumb represents death. The forefinger is symbolic of evil, the middle finger sickness, the ring finger is the symbol of sorrow, and the little finger represents the revealed. Like the Tree of Life, the fingers on both hands are in perfect balance.

The ancient Kabbalists also practiced an early version of therapeutic touch, which is still used by Kabbalists today. Three fingers of the right hand are used to channel the universe's healing energy. This technique is known as the "Spiritual Injection." We will talk more about this technique in chapter 13.

Touch is something humans and animals employ naturally. By touching each other we feel connected. We kiss, we hug, we slap each other on the backs, and we shake hands—all forms of touching.

In my opinion, shaking hands is more important that kissing. Maybe I'm getting old? I would prefer that instead of making right to right hand contact when we shake hands, we would do it Kabbalistically—right hand grasping left hand.

When both people use their right hand in the handshake, it signifies that I'm accepting the good in you and you're accepting the good in me. This gesture corresponds to the right, or positive side, of the Tree of Life.

However, if we shook hands with the right and left hand, it would be a much more meaningful gesture. We symbolically ask each other: Can you accept the shadow in me? Imagine how much more important it is to be accepted both for your faults and your strong points.

There is much power in touch. The first thing a mother does after she gives birth is touch her child. This makes the mother feel as if the child were still inside her. She can still capture that feeling of oneness she once had with her developing infant.

So when we touch each other in friendship, it signifies that we are two souls touching. And that is very important. Let's now practice a couple of healing techniques that utilize therapeutic touch.

Exercise

Sit comfortably and place your hands together in a prayerful position. This is how Christians and Hindus pray. This symbolizes the unity or balance of positive and negative energy in your body.

Next, put the point of all ten fingers near your lips to indicate a silent, listening position. Close your eyes and, in this position, begin your favorite meditation. This is a position of oneness.

In the oneness there is Allness. And in the Allness there is the answer to your health problem. Listen. If you listen closely and carefully enough, God may tell you what needs to be done.

Exercise

Stand up and place your palms together symbolizing balance. Visualize all the people of the world doing the same thing. Millions of right hands and left hands throughout the planet are placed palm together in this universal symbol of harmony.

Say the word *shalom,* meaning peace. Each time you speak this word turn in one of the four directions—East, West, North, and South. Visualize peace, health, harmony, and balance throughout the world and in yourself. See yourself possessing all these positive qualities of life.

Now end this visualization with the words: *Hakol baseder b'ezrath Hashem.* "All is in divine order with the help of God." Amen.

The Way of the Mystic

"Bestow upon me insight and understanding to penetrate and comprehend the depths of the secret mysteries of Thy Holy Word."
—Kabbalistic prayer—

In order for your healing work with the sacred tree to be successful, you are going to have to suspend your ordinary awareness of life and become like the mystic.

That's because the "tree" we will be entering is a magical one where the spirit of God can be found in its branches if we learn how to develop our spiritual eyes. Enlightenment and revelation can be experienced according to your own state of intuitive readiness.

Later in this chapter we will learn a technique called the "Mystic Trance," which teaches you how to enter a mystical state of consciousness. Before we learn it, let's discuss what mysticism is all about and gain a glimpse into the mind of the mystic.

Mysticism is nothing more than a more intensified state of consciousness than normal waking consciousness. It is neither esoteric nor strange nor fanciful. It is sublime, universal, and profoundly practical. In fact, mysticism without any practical application is worthless.

Theory must be accompanied by action. They go hand in hand. If you are just sitting on the top of that mystical mountain and not doing something helpful on earth as well, then you're simply indulging yourself.

You should be using your mystical skills in a practical way. This is pointed out in a story about Lilith, Adam's first wife. According to Kabbalah, Adam got up one morning and said to Lilith: "Honey, would you please bring me a glass of water?" Lilith shook her head and replied, "Get it yourself, Adam."

When God heard that conversation, He/She realized that this relationship wasn't going to further His/Her plan to teach the importance of union between male and female.

The Creator had foreseen that Adam was going to have a lot of responsibility in the years ahead, and he needed a helpmate. Lilith didn't want to fill that role. So God created Eve to replace Adam's first wife.

The study of Kabbalah teaches us how to discover the fire of spirituality everywhere and in everything. But this discovery also carries with it the responsibility to make the hidden light shine in our daily relationships and experiences. This is the ultimate purpose of our existence.

What you do with your knowledge of Kabbalah is important. Are you planning to imitate the ways of God in your daily life? Are you going to do things to help people?

Will you utilize your secret knowledge to promote social justice? That is the secret to entering the mystical garden. You must experience and participate in the entire world.

In a mystical state the view is different. If you are seriously ill, it is easy to get caught up in the negativity of which the medical profession is so often guilty. But if you develop mystical eyes, then you can see things in a fresh manner regardless of what your doctor has to say.

For example, my terrace is located on the nineteenth floor of a building overlooking Central Park. If I'm on my terrace and see something very beautiful, I may call up to my neighbor who lives on the third floor. I'll say, "Go to the window and see what I see."

He calls back to say, "You're crazy. All I see is another building." He would have to be on the nineteenth floor and have a terrace to see what I see.

If you move your awareness to higher level, you see things differently. Your entire psychological, emotional, and spiritual approach to life and its problems is viewed from a new dimension.

This attitude is certainly an asset for promoting health. It makes you see yourself not just as another case out of some medical textbook, but as a spiritual and eternal being.

Once you become aware that the Divine Spirit dwells within each of us, this compels us to realize that something more powerful than modern medicine is available to help restore good health.

When we pray, we are constantly adoring, praising, and loving God. These prayers express the truth, "Without God, what am I?" Yet the opposite is also true for the mystic: "Without me, what is God? We go together, we need each other. We are in partnership with God— *Shutaf Elohim*."

The mystic has a universal vision, one which compels him or her to see the presence of God in all things. The goal of the mystic is to inspire others to manifest their own spiritual natures.

The Hebrew word for God's name is *Yehovah* (YHVH). No one knows what this secret name means. As a Kabbalist, I have often thought about it. Kabbalists constantly play with numbers—*gematria*—and letters to derive secret meanings for words that appear in the *Torah*.

One day while in a mystic trance I developed this interpretation for God's mysterious name. I substituted a word that had meaning for me for each of those four Hebrew letters—*Yod, Hay, Vav, Hay* (YHVH)— that comprise the name of God.

The "*Yod*" stands for *Yirah*, which means to be in awe of everything; creation, the sun, the moon, the stars, the earth, and certainly other human beings. If it is true that God created each one of us in His/Her image, then we have to see God in every person we meet.

That's why we must observe the commandment to "Love thy neighbor as thyself." That's how we get nearer to God. This may have been the mystical meaning when Jesus said, "only through me can you go to God." He didn't mean only through him, what he meant is that God was present in all human beings and we have to recognize that.

The Hebrew letter "*Hay*" stands for *Henani*, which means "I'm ready. I'm here and I'm ready, God, just tell me what to do." You experience the Creator when you say this word, which Abraham uttered when God called him. Later Moses repeated that same word. The chances are that every great rabbi or guru who establishes contact with the Lord has uttered that word.

The "*Vav*" stands for *Vedue*, which means confession. The way to get to God is by confession. Confession means to go over the day's events. It is not so much about confessing your shameful secrets to a priest or rabbi. It's about confessing to yourself because you're the only one who knows if you've done something.

The letter "*Vav*" further symbolizes to me confession to the Heavenly Father/Mother. It signifies the Father/Mother and child relationship that we have with the Lord. Even the way this Hebrew letter is written—it's a straight line going up and down—suggests the straight, open, and honest relationship that we need to have with God. There is no hiding from God.

The final letter "*Hay*," suggests life to me. When we finish our meditation on God's name by saying *Henani*—I am ready—we are ready to bring new life and health into being. We are more open, more accepting, more loving, more joyous, and more peaceful.

Now you see the magical way in which mystics enter the gates of wisdom. There is never just one way to enter these gates, but a multiplicity of approaches.

When you begin your healing work with the Tree of Life, you may find that there are seventy ways that the spheres, which line the cosmic tree, can speak to you. What you will need to do is find the gateway that resonates in your heart. That is the way of the mystic.

Try to keep in mind that you cannot live on the mystical level all the time. There are some enlightened masters who always stay on this mountain, but for most of us it's too easy to get hung up there and ignore other less mystical necessities of our lives. Remember the image of Jacob's Ladder. The angels are always going up and down, not remaining in one place.

One of the mystical ways to reach God is through "confession." The following exercise, which I often suggest to my Kabbalah students to teach them how to use confession to attain inner peace, will help you arise in the morning with a feeling of peace. This exercise needs to be done at night just before you fall asleep.

Exercise

Lay on your back and close your eyes. Visualize a white screen and a slide projector. On the right side of the screen is a list of all the things you did during the day that were pleasing to you, pleasing to the people around you, and, therefore, pleasing to God.

On the left side of the screen look at the list of all the things that you didn't do or shouldn't have done. Look at this list and accept it. Confess to yourself all the things you did wrong. "I'm sorry, I did this but this is me." And if another human was hurt by something that you said or did, call that person in the morning to say you are sorry.

Now silently repeat this mantra. *"In His hands I deposit my soul and my body. Awake or asleep, God is with me."*

Visualize God waiting for you to put your soul and your body into His/Her keeping for the night. Do not fear. Then repeat another mantra: *"Adonai le veloh erah."* God is with me. I do not fear. Then go to sleep.

The Mystic Trance

Tree of Life pathwork requires much use of your intuitive talents and imaginative powers. Techniques such as meditation, visualization, and prayer are often required in order to enter that state of higher consciousness known as the "mystical state."

Ritual is also important in attaining this trance state. In fact, ritual is as important in Kabbalah as it is in the practice of magic. In magic, however, the metaphysician gets into the proper mindset through the use of ritualistic tools such as wands, gowns, swords, and other objects. These tools serve to enhance the practitioner's level of concentration.

In Kabbalah, however, we don't use wands or other tools. To attain a mystical state of consciousness, Kabbalists use other methods, among them are relaxation techniques, meditation, deep breathing, dancing, singing, and chanting.

Much like Zen, in the Hassidic tradition, answers are not the goal. The moment you have an answer, things are no longer spontaneous. Instead, you try to comprehend God with your heart, not your mind.

This is the key to entering a mystic trance. You must not let intellect or skepticism interfere with your efforts to heighten your spiritual powers. You must sense the Divine intuitively and be ready to receive.

Nor should you discuss the feelings associated with the mystic trance or its results with anyone. Trying to talk about a mystical experience defuses this emotion-charged state of consciousness. You are attempting to raise power, and discussion only serves to dissipate it.

Many Kabbalists practice prolonged meditative silence to attain a mystic trance state, while others prefer more action-oriented techniques like song, chanting, and even dance.

The following meditative technique will help you experience the "mystic trance." My Kabbalah students have found it useful for bringing God fully into their awareness and inducing a high level of concentration.

I often use the symbol of Jacob's ladder to help my students achieve this trance state. In the Biblical story, Jacob dreamed of a ladder with the angels of the Lord going up and down.

> *And behold a ladder was set up on the earth, and the top of it reached into heaven; and behold the angels of God ascending and descending on it.*
>
> —Genesis 28:12

Exercise

Find a quiet place where you will not be disturbed. Stand up and close your eyes. Do the breathing exercise described in chapter 3 (page 61).

Next, visualize a golden ladder connected from earth to heaven. Start climbing that ladder, slowly, one rung at a time. Breathe deeply as you climb. Move upwards as high as you can go. In your mind's eye, see the beautiful angels flying around you. They are there to help in case you should stumble or fall.

As you climb, think of the Psalm:

> *Unto Thee, O Lord, do I lift up my soul*
>
> —Psalm 25:1

Or you may recite the mantra *Yod, Hay, Vav, Hay*—the letters which form the sacred name *Yehovah.* You may even substitute your own favorite mantra if you so wish.

Keep repeating those letters as you climb each rung of the ladder. Feel your love for God and His/Her love for you as you climb higher and higher. The higher you climb, the deeper your trance becomes as you move closer to the light of God.

Keep repeating the letters *Yod, Hay, Vav, Hay.* Once you have reached the top of the ladder pause and listen. You are now ready to do anything that God wants you to do. You are also ready to enter the Tree of Life.

If you don't like heights and are not comfortable climbing ladders, then try this Kabbalistic practice known as "riding the letters" to help you fall into a mystical trance.

Instead of climbing a ladder, you will visualize the letters *Yod, Hay, Vav, Hay* appearing before you, because God is always in front of you.

Exercise

Sit back, relax, and imagine a blank screen before you. The four letters *Yod, Hay, Vav, Hay* are projected on this screen. Examine each letter one at a time.

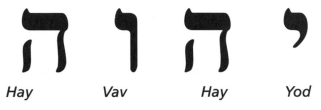

| Hay | Vav | Hay | Yod |

Figure 6

Visualize the *Yod*. Look at it. Think about it. What does it look like? What images does it present to you? Is it standing still or dancing? Isolate it from the other letters and enter into a personal relationship with it.

Now take a deep breath and visualize the other three letters the same way. Next, observe each of these individual letters as they now join together, unifying with each other to spell God's Holy Name. You are now like King David who wrote in one of his psalms: "I have placed *Yod, Hay, Vav, Hay* before me at all times."

Breathe the Sacred Name of *Yehovah* into the areas of your body where you are feeling pain or discomfort. Fill your head with the Sacred Name, or your torso, your stomach, your legs or your heart—wherever you may feel the need for healing.

These letters, which spell one of God's many secret names, are now within you. They permeate and surround you with the Divine Presence. You are God, God is You. "*I am ready, I am ready, I am ready for a healing.*"

The Sounds of Music

Some Kabbalists attain an ecstatic state by singing or humming a wordless melody over and over again. This repetitive, wordless melody is called a *nigun*. Others mystics enter a trance state by singing sacred songs.

For such musically oriented mystics, song is considered preferable to contemplative meditation or even prayer for attaining an ecstatic state of mind.

One of Hassidism's most learned rabbis, Rabbi Nachman of Breslov, the great grandson of the Baal Shem Tov, believed that singing and dancing were equal to study and silent meditation for attaining a mystical state. He always emphasized such joyful and spontaneous meditation.

If you are not comfortable with singing, there are plenty of tapes and CDs featuring sacred music that you can listen to, but the music must be vibrant. It must resonate with sound and power. It has been scientifically proven that music can affect the brain's alpha waves, which are associated with deep relaxed, meditative states. The Kabbalists have understood this principle for centuries.

So whether you want to sing a *nigun* or put on your headphones, let the music enliven and excite you. You want to build up your reservoir of psychic energy.

Chanting

Devotional chanting is a form of meditation that vocally celebrates the Divine. It is also another powerful way to attain a state of trance. Chanting has been described by Swami Sivananda as "melting the heart, filling the mind with purity, and generating divine love and harmony."

Almost every spiritual tradition incorporates devotional chanting, including Kabbalah. Most orthodox Jews wrap themselves in prayer shawls and chant. Muslims chant from the tops of minarets and Hindus intone sacred mantras.

Many Kabbalists like to chant the introductory verses to the Psalms. Some chant the holy letters of the Sacred Name—*Yad, Hay, Vav, Hay*. The chanting of the Bible is also a form of sacred meditation.

If you chant, do so with enthusiasm. Beat a drum if you want to like the Native Americans do. This is one of the most powerful tools for transforming consciousness, with the power to open our hearts, heal our bodies, and shift our realities.

Good Vibrations

"Vibrating" the Divine names of God along with the names of various Archangels is another trance-inducing method that continues to be used by Kabbalists.

Each letter comprising one of the holy names of God or the names of the four Archangels is slowly pronounced. Y…E…H…O…V…A… H. Feel the letters vibrating as you pronounce them. M…i…c…h…. a…e…l, G…a…b…r…i…a…l, A…r…i…e…l, R…a…f…a…e…l.

When you are "vibrating" these letters, close your eyes, raise your eyes under your closed lids and "look" at the letters. Visualize the *Shekinah* descending from heaven and bringing white healing light with her.

Visualize the light passing through the letters and into places in your body where you need healing. Let this healing energy build up within you. Feel health and balance being restored deep inside you.

Touched by Angels

When visualizing Archangels to reach a trance state, it can be helpful to also visualize the colors associated with these celestial visitors. Gold, for example, is the color of the gown that Michael wears. Red is usually associated with Gabriel who represents strength. Gold and silver are the colors of Ariel's robes as he leads us toward God, and green is the color associated with Rafael, the angel of healing.

As your meditation deepens, imagine the Archangels surrounding you. They are huge, and their faces are hidden under their cowls because the light of God, which shines from them, might blind you.

Feel the love and healing power emanating from all of them. At the same time, feel the *Shekinah* shining upon you. Now, as you approach your trance state, continue to let go of all your tensions and summon Gabriel, the healing angel. Ask him to help you with your health problem. The following exercise will help you summon Gabriel's help.

Exercise

Close your eyes and take long, deep breaths. Picture yourself seated in a beautiful landscape of your own choosing: a valley, a mountainside, a knoll overlooking the ocean. This can be a place you have visited or one that only exists in your imagination.

Look! There in the distance is Gabriel slowly approaching you. His green robe covers his body and most of his face, but you can see the bright healing light, which bathes him, streaming out from under his robe.

Slowly, this healing angel approaches you. He seems to be floating. His feet do not touch the ground. Now the archangel stands before you. He asks why you summoned him. With humility and gratitude you explain why you have called him and where you may need healing.

The archangel reaches out his hand and touches you. You feel the healing power of his hand flow through you. Feel it as if his hand is really touching you. You are being healed through the power of God who works through his beloved angels. Bask in this energy. Stay with it as long as you can.

Fasting

A mystic trance can also be attained by fasting for two or three days. Kabbalists who go on such prolonged fasts avoid sexual activity and refrain from impure or destructive thoughts.

While fasting, mystics often sing spiritual songs, and read scripture like the Psalms. Quite often these fasts not only lead to heightened states of consciousness, but also result in visions.

Before you embark on any prolonged fasting, make certain you consult with your primary physician first. If you decide to fast, pay close attention to any images you may receive during the fasting process. These images or visions can often provide important clues to your state of health.

Power Prayers

Another way to heighten your state of consciousness and enter a mystic trance is through prayer. Don't be content with the recital of fixed prayers. Bring your heart into it. Make it sing. As you pray, feel a sense of expansion. Feel enthusiasm, love, and joy.

According to the Baal Shem Tov, "if you become one with prayer, you become one with God." What a wonderful way to enter the Tree of Life—with prayer on your lips. With prayer, the soul flies high like one of the angels.

Dance, Dance, Dance

Ritual dance can also induce ecstasy and raise consciousness. Dance has been used by everyone from the "Whirling Dervishes" in the Sufi spiritual tradition to the Hassidic Jews. Dance helps us to bypass our everyday states of consciousness. It builds and releases energy, putting us into a different state of mind.

Dance to the image of the sacred letters YHVH or the four elements of life—fire, water, air, or earth. You don't need any particular dance skills. Just let go and bring all your consciousness and imagination into this activity.

Get a Little Crazy

According to Kabbalistic tradition, if you are not involved in silent meditation, then you should try to utilize every part of you to enter a mystic trance. That's why the Hassidim dance, sway, sing, stomp their feet, and clap their hands during many of their religious services.

To outsiders, they may even look crazy. But you have to be crazy sometimes. Craziness can lead to the path of ecstasy. Crazy simply means being alive—I'm not like I normally am—I'm not sitting at my desk and playing the role of a gentleman.

Personally I don't think God likes gentlemen or ladies. He/She likes people who have feelings and express them. I guess that's why I so often find myself arguing with God!

By now I think you have a pretty good idea of what it takes to get out of your ordinary everyday consciousness and into that state of mystical trance. The secret is innovation and enthusiasm. Open your heart and mind to a different way of doing things.

Once you have purified yourself, worked on preparing body, mind, and soul to receive the healing light, and entered a higher state of consciousness, you are now ready to proceed to that extraordinary place known as the Tree of Life.

The Tree of Life

"Keep the way of the Tree of Life."
—Genesis 3:24—

The Tree of Life is a spiritual map that helps to explain God's role in the universe and how we fit into the scheme of things. This sacred tree consists of ten *sefiroth,* or spheres, that are considered a secret key to the reason and purpose of existence.

One of the simplest ways to visualize the Tree of Life is to view it as three pillars. The right pillar represents our positive inclinations or impulses—the *yetzer hatov.* The left pillar symbolizes our negative inclinations—the *yetzer harah.*

The middle pillar is generally considered neutral. The spheres lining this middle section of the tree gain their significance from the other globes to which they are connected via twenty-two lines called "paths." These paths correspond to the twenty-two letters of the Hebrew alphabet.

Kabbalists refer to the ten spheres and twenty-two paths as the "thirty-two paths of wisdom." It is through a study of these spheres and paths that we can learn how the creative Source of Life manifests itself.

To help you understand this order of creation, imagine a jagged flash of lightning zigzagging down the tree from one side to the other. This lightning flash originates at the first sphere, the Crown, *Kether,* located on top of the tree and representing the highest divinity.

The lightning bolt then zigzags downward to the right and then left activating various spheres or globes until it works its way down to strike the tenth and final sphere, the Kingdom, *Malkut.* This globe represents the final result of creation and its purpose—to establish the Kingdom of God on earth.

There are many meanings attributed to these ten spheres of light, but our focus is on how they can help to bring about health and healing.

What the spheres are not, however, are fortune-telling devices or some kind of a divining rod.

They cannot predict the future, despite the fact that tarot and other divinatory systems are based upon the Tree of Life. However, these spheres certainly do have a story to tell us—the story of our souls.

The Tree of Life blooms because it is in harmony. It teaches us a lesson about the great value of staying in balance. Harmony comes when resistance is faced with love instead of confronted with opposition.

We are harmonized to life's tune when we accept the rain as a sister to the sun and use the wake of the storm as a quiet time to mobilize our inner perspective.

From your reading of chapter 1 you have learned that the spheres, which are connected to each other via "branches," often contain opposite characteristics, yet they remain in dynamic equilibrium.

As was discussed earlier (chapter 1, see "Staying Balanced"), this is one of the key messages of the Tree of Life—the dynamics of opposing forces. To review briefly, let's look at the spheres of Compassion and Judgment. Although directly linked they have opposite traits.

The result of their union, however, is a third sphere called Beauty. It becomes clear that when judgment, or severity, is tempered by compassion, or mercy, the result is spiritual understanding or beauty.

Similarly, although the spheres of Wisdom and Knowledge have opposing meanings, it is by bringing them into harmony that we gain enlightenment. And although the sphere of Victory emphasizes ego, and the sphere of Glory in Splendour emphasizes humility, when in balance they strengthen Foundation.

According to Kabbalah, balance is always the road to spiritual wholeness, and the harmony, which results from balance, is our greatest defense against disease. Attaining balance in our body, mind, and soul energy centers is also a powerful weapon to reverse ill health.

In order to create such balance, you must remember the words of the Buddha (see chapter 1) who spoke about the importance of being aware and awake. Applied to your quest for health, the Buddha's words mean that you must always remain conscious of the *entirety* of your being.

Now, before we begin our climb among the branches of the cosmic tree, let's first make certain that you're properly oriented—that you recognize *where you are.*

Let's say, for example, that you live out of town and you want to come to visit me. I give you instructions on how to get here. All of a sudden you call me up, and you say, "Rabbi, I'm lost." The first question I will ask you is "Where are you?"

And that was the first question that God asked Adam when he was hiding after eating the forbidden fruit. "Where are you?" The Lord knew exactly where Adam was hiding. The question pertained not only to Adam, but to all the generations of men and women who would follow. "*Where are you?*"

If you know where you are, then someone can help you. Knowing where you are is vital if you wish to recover from whatever ails you. It is, perhaps, the most important question you need to answer; where are you on your life journey that may have resulted in your disease in the first place?

Using the metaphor of the highway again, think of health as a beautiful highway. Sickness is like getting lost on that highway. First you have to get out of cruise control and become aware that you somehow managed to get off that road. Next, you must become absolutely committed to the idea of returning to that highway of perfect health, and not simply content to drive along life's secondary roads to get to your destination. This is where you're going to need a roadmap called The Tree of Life.

Reading the Map

Okay, let's take a look at our roadmap and become familiar with the kingdom we're going to be traveling through. The roadmap is shaped like a giant tree.

When we are doing healing work we need to align this tree properly with our body. This means that the right side of the tree corresponds to our right arm, hands, and legs, and the left side to our left arm, hand, and leg (see Fig. 7).

The spheres of Wisdom, Compassion, and Victory correspond to the right side of your body, while the spheres of Knowledge, Judgment, and Glory in Splendour correspond to the left side of your body.

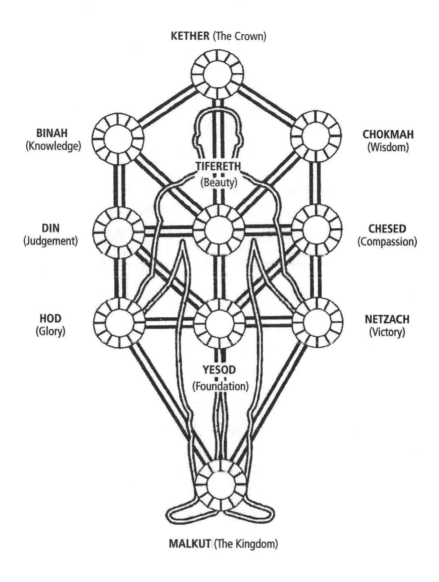

KETHER (The Crown)

BINAH
(Knowledge)

CHOKMAH
(Wisdom)

TIFERETH
(Beauty)

DIN
(Judgement)

CHESED
(Compassion)

HOD
(Glory)

NETZACH
(Victory)

YESOD
(Foundation)

MALKUT (The Kingdom)

Figure 7: Correspondences Between Human Body and Tree of Life

At the top of the map you will see a sphere called the Crown, *Kether*. The Crown is the entrance way to the Tree of Life, and the holy light that shines through all the other spheres or globes. It corresponds to the head in the human body.

Over the centuries the Crown has been given many different divine names. It has been called Ra by the ancient Egyptians; Manitou by Native Americans; Brahma by the Buddhists; Allah by the Muslims; and Krishna by the Hindus. In yoga, it corresponds to the crown chakra.

The Crown represents the highest divinity—all that God is as a metaphysical concept. And since, according to Kabbalistic tradition, you and God are always in a partnership, then the Crown also represents you.

This is the crown to your kingdom, which is your body, mind, and soul. Once you decide to enter the Tree of Life and wear the crown, then it becomes your responsibility to maintain your kingdom and make more than superficial repairs should things break down.

Certainly if there is a problem in your kingdom you will get expert help first—a doctor or some other specialist. But then you'll launch your own personal investigation and try to get to the bottom of things to make certain it never happens again.

This is what I believe Rabbi Hillel meant when he said those three beautiful things: "If I am not for myself, who will be? If I am for myself only, what am I? If not now, when?"

In other words, if I'm not for myself, then I can't do what I'm supposed to do for myself, which is to create peace, health, and harmony within my kingdom. Nobody else can really do that for me. Only I can discover the deeper mental, physical, or spiritual reasons that may have led to the onset of my disorder.

The Hebrew word for peace is *shalom*. And peace comes from harmony in your kingdom. You must learn to temper judgment with compassion, rely on feelings as well as thoughts, meld wisdom with knowledge, and always strive for beauty in your life. These are some of the ways you can attain such peace and harmony.

Continuing down our cosmic roadmap, you will see that the Crown is connected to the spheres of Wisdom and Knowledge. All three of these spheres form a triad, which corresponds to the head in the human body.

The sphere of Wisdom, *Chokmah,* is sometimes also known as "Spiritual Will." According to Kabbalah, this sphere suggests the value of self-appraisal—the need to check in with yourself to see if you have grown any wiser since yesterday.

Remember the psycho/spiritual checkup you took earlier in this book? (See chapter 5, page 74.) That is the idea expressed here; the need for "in-sight" or looking within. Wisdom is the highway that leads to the sphere called Knowledge.

Knowledge, *Binah*, is a sphere which is sometimes also identified as Understanding. Where Wisdom is a dynamic force, Knowledge or Understanding is more passive—through wisdom comes knowledge.

The Kabbalists considered Wisdom to be a more positive attribute than Knowledge because of the Biblical story of King Solomon who, when asked by God what he wanted the most, replied "Wisdom."

As a modern interpreter of Kabbalah, this is one concept with which I disagree somewhat. I don't think we should pit wisdom against knowledge or explain them in opposite terms. Instead, we should put more emphasis on the relationship between the two.

Wisdom is the wife and Knowledge is the husband. It is a partnership. Like a husband and wife, they must learn how to live together in harmony. They must support each other and talk to each other.

Moving down our map a bit further, we arrive at a destination called Compassion, *Chesed*, corresponding to the right arm on the human body. Compassion, you will note, is connected by a road that leads directly to Judgment, *Din*.

Compassion, also known as Mercy, Loving Kindness, and Benevolence, is considered a superior quality by Kabbalists because it allows one to forgive himself or herself, others, and even life itself, regardless of what adversity it may bring—including poor health.

Much of this thinking is also based on the Bible. The Bible is filled with accounts of how God's heart was softened against the Israelites and filled with mercy despite all their transgressions against Him.

In Hebrew, the sphere of Compassion is sometimes called *Gedulah*, which means greatness or magnificence. It's obvious that to the Kabbalists, Compassion is way up there on the cosmic scale.

Directly across the map from Compassion is the sphere called Judgment, also sometimes known as "Strength," "Severity," "Justice," "Discipline," and "Restraint." It corresponds to the left arm. This is the sphere of power with no compassion.

This globe is not as negative as it may sound. Without the strong arm of Judgment, Compassion or Mercy can come to signify the idealist who succumbs to folly and cowardliness.

Justice defends and corrects. It prevents virtue from turning into a vice. This is another Kabbalistic lesson that emphasizes the importance of keeping things in balance.

There is a wonderful rest stop en route from Compassion to Judgment. It is called Beauty, or *Tifereth*. Another name for this sphere is Harmony.

Positioned near the exact center of the Tree of Life, Beauty is the link between the upper branches of the tree—the metaphysical center—and the lower branches of the tree containing spheres related to personality and the bodily senses. Beauty is the heart of the Tree of Life, and, not surprisingly, corresponds to the human heart.

This heart of your kingdom beats with joy when Compassion and Judgment are in balance. Beauty is where the light from the Crown starts to come alive. This sphere reminds us that the source of beauty is in kindness, which occurs when severity, or judgment, is tempered with mercy.

A little further down the map we now come to Victory, *Netzach*. This sphere, also called "Endurance," "Fortitude," and "Ambition," is connected by a road to the sphere known as Glory in Splendour, *Hod*.

The sphere of Victory—or Triumph, as it is sometimes also called—represents a feeling of firmness. That is why it corresponds to the hips and legs of the human body.

Victory is considered a positive attribute as long as its celebration isn't excessive—especially in the arena of sexual conquest. Any overemphasis on Victory—and this includes excessive gratification of our baser natures—must be balanced by the sphere of Glory in Splendour located just across the road. Glory symbolizes humility and indicates that man must not glory in the ego, but in growth.

As a modern Kabbalist, my explanation of the sphere of Victory is that it represents the typical American male who made it. "I'm the self-made man," he boastfully asserts.

What follows when he says that? God speaks to him through the sphere of Glory in Splendour. If this typical American male bothered to pay any attention, he would hear God saying to him, "Don't glory in your victory; don't glory in your ego."

But, of course, like so many of us, this American male often fails to listen. Instead, this so-called victorious man lives a life of lavish spending and excess carnal activity. Sooner or later, of course, such a lifestyle will catch up with him.

It is likely that he—or she—will pay the price for excess with psychological or physical illness—broken relationships, loneliness. Who knows what can come about as a result of such excessive behavior?

To be truly victorious we must resolve the civil war between our positive and negative inclinations that rages within each of us. We must accept and integrate both of these inclinations and act with God in all things.

That is the purpose of the sphere called Glory in Splendour. It always reminds us that we should not celebrate the ego and let our unchecked emotions turn us into fools. Instead, we must glory in growth and master our minds as well as our baser nature.

On the lower part of our roadmap, we now arrive at a sphere called Foundation, or *Yesod*. This sphere is sometimes referred to as the "Vehicle of Life," because it corresponds to the reproductive organs. The phallus is often a symbol of *Yesod*.

Foundation, which provides a framework for the world of matter, urges us to say "yes" to life in a positive manner. It discourages an overactive libido and encourages "giving birth" to a new day or a new child with positive thoughts in mind and always in the name of the Divine.

Foundation is the birth child of Victory and Glory in Splendour. But the foundation cannot be a steady one if Victory is not balanced by Glory. The message in this grouping of Victory, Glory in Splendor, and Foundation is that for sound physical and emotional health, our reproductive organs need to be used in a loving and positive manner, and not as a tool of conquest.

At the very bottom of our map is a sphere called Kingdom, *Malkut*. "Nobility," "Sovereignty," and "Leadership" are other names often attributed to this sphere. This tenth and last *sefira* represents man's final, ultimate mastery over life's challenges by his union with God.

Malkut represents the Kingdom of life—the sum of all the lessons we have learned from our travels through the sacred tree. It is the "Kingdom of the Father spread upon the Earth," that St. Thomas spoke of in his Gospel. In our human body, this globe represents our sensations.

The need for all of us to create the Kingdom of God within ourselves is the basic message of this sphere. It is no mapmaker's error that the Crown and the Kingdom are on opposite ends of the sacred tree.

Rather, the message is perfectly clear; The entry to your kingdom begins when you put on the crown, and ends as a gateway to the better understanding of yourself and the world.

Now might be a good time for you to put down your roadmap for a moment, and consider all that you have learned so far. You might also want to start asking yourself questions such as:

"Where have I come from and where do I want to go?" "What mistakes do I need to correct so that I don't make another wrong turn off the highway to good health?"

This is what is so important about working with the sacred tree. It heightens our transcendental outlook. It hones our intuitive insights. It clarifies existing conflicts of thoughts, feelings, and actions.

Above all, the cosmic tree always serves to remind us what we must do and think in order to stay on the path of wholeness. It points the way to that highway called perfect health.

Triads

I'd like to take a brief moment to point out another interesting way for you to read your roadmap. Besides thinking about the Tree of Life as three pillars, you may also wish to view it as three separate triangles or triads (see Fig. 8).

These three triads, or tricycles, also correspond to the human body. The first triad is comprised of the Crown, Wisdom, and Knowledge. The spheres in this triad essentially correspond to our metaphysical and spiritual life. It represents the spirit within us, as well as the spirit without— universal life, or the intelligence of the world.

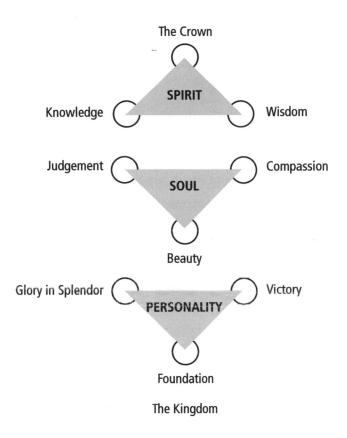

Figure 8: The Three Triads

The second triad consists of the spheres of Compassion, Judgment, and Beauty. These spheres generally represent moral character. This is the region of the soul or our emotions. This grouping suggests that the source of beauty rests in kindness and God's grace.

The spheres of Victory, Glory in Splendour, and Foundation make up the third triad. This cluster of spheres corresponds to our personality or senses—how the soul enters the physical form. The body, feelings, and subconscious thoughts are all associated with this triad.

For those of you who prefer this way of visualizing the Tree of Life, let me offer you a metaphor which will help to sharpen this image. Have you ever seen one of those three-legged kitchen tables that our grandmothers used to own?

Suppose you owned one of those old tables. One morning you came home and a leg on the table was loose or broken. You could no longer eat off that table because it had become too shaky.

The same holds true for these three triads. If a sphere in any one of them is ignored or neglected, the entire cluster becomes shaky. This can only mean problems in health or in other areas of your life.

Before concluding our overview of the Tree of Life, keep in mind that this diagram of the Sacred Tree is designed to give you the insight, the wisdom, and the power to realize that each of you has within you your own Tree of Life.

Always remind yourself of that. To reinforce this image, you may wish to repeat this affirmation:

I am the Tree of Life. Here is my Crown. My ears represent Wisdom and Knowledge. They dwell together and speak to me when I am open to listening and learning.

Compassion and Judgment are my arms, to be used to embrace my brother. Putting my hands together I am whole, the positive and the negative before me. My heart is tempered by Victory and Glory.

At the center of my chest, over my heart, is Beauty. I am moved by the beauty of life around me, the beauty that is God. I stand with the support of the Foundation, upon the Kingdom of God.

The following exercise will help familiarize you with the ten spheres and will help you to establish a close personal relationship with this sacred tree.

Exercise

Find a comfortable and quiet place where you will not be disturbed. Do some breathing exercises and try to relax. Now, visualize the Tree of Life. Visualize the lightning pattern in Figure 2.

Focus your attention on that pattern. See the lightning flash of creation as it strikes sphere one, then sphere two and so forth. With each lightning strike, try to identify any qualities of the globe that remind you of yourself.

The qualities can be either positive or negative. What are you feeling as you see the lightning strike each sphere? Are you feeling upset? What is it that is causing this upset? Is this sphere touching something deep within you that needs to be addressed? Meditate on this.

Contemplate the relationship between the spheres, the paths that connect them, or anything else about the tree that strikes a responsive chord. Dwell in the tree for a while.

Follow the lightning flash to the bottom of the tree and then reverse its course. Follow the zigzag bolts of lightning from the bottom to top. Repeat this pattern several times. Up and down, down and up. Don't get stuck in any one place.

When this meditation is finished, repeat the following mantra: "*Help me transform my grief to purpose, my sickness to health, for the sake of God, for the sake of humanity, and for my own sake. My soul still has things to do in life.*"

The Healing Tree

"…And on either side of the river, was a Tree of Life, which bare twelve manners of fruits, and yielded her fruit every month; and the leaves of the fruit were for the healing of all nations."
—Revelation 22:2—

Now that you understand the basic pattern of the Tree of Life, we are going to begin climbing the tree so that we can apply the lessons of the ten *sefiroth* to the healing of our mind, body, and soul.

In every religious tradition there are always two aspects, the seen and the hidden. We are now in that world of hidden things. We are in a world of imagination and intuition where the twenty-four-hour clock is temporarily suspended and only angels dwell.

The Tree of Life is a mystical place where we must learn how to relate to symbols and try to understand their meaning in order to draw Divine power into our lives and attain a subsequent sense of well-being.

As you read this chapter, remember that our pathwork through the Tree of Life is only a preliminary tour laced with just a few general examples. It would be impossible within the scope of this book to list all ailments that unfortunately afflict us and how the tree may be used for healing.

So it is up to you to take what you have learned here and adapt it to your own particular situation. Let this be your starting point. Now you must go on to consider the meaning, the purpose, and the wisdom of what you learn, and use that knowledge as a bridge to help you reach your goal of good health and total healing. With all that said and done, let us now begin our travels through the sacred tree.

The First Triad: Head and Neck Problems

We now enter the first triad on the Tree of Life: Crown, Wisdom, and

Knowledge. This triad corresponds to the top of the human body, especially the head and neck areas.

For many of us, the head is where we often experience various physical pains and emotional illness, from the simple headache to serious problems such as depression.

If your health concern is related to the cranium or skull area, I suggest the underlying reason for this problem is that one of the three spheres in this triad is out of harmony.

Do you know the saying, "It's all in your head?" It's an expression that was borrowed from Kabbalah. We sometimes use it jokingly to suggest an imaginary illness, but it has very serious significance. According to Kabbalah, what goes on in the head can most definitely affect the rest of the body.

Therefore, if you are experiencing discomfort in this part of the body—and that includes the neck and upper back area—your meditation should focus on the spheres of this triad.

After first consulting with a physician, your next step should be to set aside some time for quiet meditation. It is during these silent moments that you need to examine your spiritual life and your relationship with the Divine Self. Is the pain or other discomfort you are feeling a result of pent-up anger, or something having to do with work?

Could your ailment have feelings of aloneness and separation from God as its root? It is questions like these that you should contemplate while meditating on the spheres of this triad.

Pain in the head may also stem from depression. Think about what is going on in your life that may be causing such feelings. Over the long years that I've worked as a psychotherapist, I've become convinced that many of my patients' physical ailments are connected to feelings of worthlessness—"who needs me?"

Depression often manifests itself when our minds receive the message: "Who wants me?" "What am I doing here?" "I might as well get sick and die." This attitude can then lead to a multitude of physical ailments.

If you are feeling depressed, meditating upon the Crown sphere will open yourself to spiritual energy. This energy is almost certain to give you the wisdom, the understanding, and the insight that you are not alone in the universe.

By meditating on the Crown, the ultimate symbol of our partnership with God, you may even hear the Creator say: "There's nothing I can do without you."

Try to remember how often you may have received the message that there is nothing you could do without God and also, how much you needed God. But now that you know something about the nature of mystical thinking, you are aware that there is also nothing that God can do without us. So you are really never alone. You are always wanted by God.

During meditation try to hear God's words. If you listen closely enough, I'm almost positive that you will hear Him/Her say, "I need you." And once you hear those words you will have a reason to live.

Not only have you discovered a friend, but also now you have a purpose and a job to do—to work in partnership with God toward your healing. I guarantee that repeated meditation on the Crown will take you further along your path to emotional healing than all the medication in the world.

Peace of Mind

Meditating on the Crown can also help eliminate much psychological distress by creating peace of mind. Since the Crown is also the symbol for your kingdom here on earth—your body—as well as God's Kingdom above, this awareness will help make you feel more secure by helping you to realize that you are the master of your own domain.

You will now understand that you are the captain of your ship. You can say to yourself, "I know who I am and I know what God has guided me to do. He has appointed me to rule my own kingdom."

Knowing that you rule a kingdom will help to lessen your aggressive tendencies. You no longer have to go around conquering any other kingdoms. You now have your own domain to manage. Peace therefore replaces aggression and tension is reduced.

Generally, we tend to relate to others with an attitude of someone intent on proving himself superior to the rest of the population: "My car is better than your car," or "my house is more beautiful than your house, therefore I'm better than you" and so on.

But as the crown head of your own kingdom, you no longer need to play that kind of game. You have your own responsibilities and plenty of work to do to carry them out.

This can lead not only to a more peaceful and relaxed state of mind, which is always conducive to good mental health, but also, since running your kingdom is such a busy job, it will help to keep your mind off your various health problems.

Will Power

I'd like to suggest that while you are meditating on the Crown, you focus your mental energy on developing the will to live. Theory and practice are useless without will.

Usually, the first thing a person who suffers pain or discomfort does is go seek out some remedy—Tums to soothe an upset stomach or aspirin for a cold. But I believe that in order to best soothe your pain, you must first focus on girding up your will power so that it can overcome the usual Doubting Thomas attitude of the ego which can slow down healing.

One way to increase your will power is to have an honest talk with your Divine partner while in meditation. Express all your troubles. Tell God about your needs, regrets, and desires. In other words, connect with spirit. This will help give you will power and the purpose you need to effect a quick healing.

Wisdom

For any kind of discomfort in the head area, you should also meditate on the spheres of Wisdom and Knowledge. According to Kabbalistic thinking, these spheres are also associated with understanding, awareness, and purpose.

Awareness of the Great Healer can lead to *purpose*. And once you have a clear understanding of your purpose, which is to be full of joy, peace, and health, then you are well on the road to well-being.

So remain aware. Listen closely with your spiritual ears and you may hear the sphere of Wisdom speaking to you. She is telling you to become awake to the fact that the body, mind, and soul are all equally part of your kingdom. These spheres are so alive that if we use our spiritual eyes, we might even come to recognize them as individuals.

"The mind is an individual, the body is an individual, and the soul is an individual," Wisdom is whispering to you. "Each has its own peculiar traits and unique personalities. And they all carry the sparks of God."

Wisdom cautions you that any one of these sparks of life is likely to do a bit of complaining if they don't like the way you are running your kingdom. If you are more involved in making money than tending to your intellectual growth, for example, then the mind begins to complain: "I was created to contain some wisdom," she scolds, "and you're more involved in making money.

"That's fine," the mind continues, "and I know it's going to make your body more comfortable. But what about me? I'm empty." That's where the expression, "empty-headed," comes from. Something is missing upstairs.

Have you been leading an empty-headed lifestyle? If after honest self-evaluation the answer is yes, you may have discovered a key to why you are having psychological, emotional, or even physical problems in the cranial area. If you're not certain, then take a psycho/spiritual checkup.

Knowledge

If you listen closely with your spiritual ears, you may also hear Knowledge speaking to you during your meditation on the head area. Knowledge is also associated with intelligence and the intellect.

Kabbalists believe that ignoring education can result in ignorance, which puts you into an imbalanced state of mind. In fact, ignorance is considered to be one of the greatest sins. That is why in Jewish tradition there is such an emphasis placed upon education.

Knowledge is quite important whether you are feeling well, or trying to heal yourself or others. If you are ill, it is incumbent upon you to do your own research into the problem beyond what a doctor may tell you.

You might research the problem on the Internet, visit the public library, or join some support group. God makes many healing tools available to us—not just miracles—and you have to be knowledgeable to make the best use of these tools.

The Hebrew word for knowledge is *binah*. The letter "b" can also stand for *bereshet*, which means creation, or *barukha*, the Hebrew word for blessing. Thus knowledge can *create* healing. It is also a *blessing*, because without it you cannot be a truly wise ruler of your kingdom.

The Crown, Wisdom, and Knowledge represent the head, right ear, and left ear which all connect to the eyes—especially the intuitive and spiritual "third eye."

If Wisdom and Knowledge are not in harmony, you will not be able to "see" and the Crown will not be able to function. And what kingdom can survive if the ruler is incapacitated?

With all three of these spheres properly integrated, you will be able to do the right thing to maintain or improve your health. You'll be able to see God in everything and everybody—including the God in you—and this will not only lead to a peaceful state of mind, but also to harmony and balance.

Keep the head in balance and it will also be easier for you to bring the rest of your body into harmony. What a wonderful way to maintain health or start your healing journey—with Crown, Wisdom, and Knowledge all in perfect equilibrium.

The Second Triad: Coronary Problems

If you suffer from heart problems, you should be paying attention to the spheres comprising the second triad, Compassion, Judgment, and Beauty. This triad corresponds with the emotions and the soul. In the human body, Beauty represents the heart.

In order for Beauty—the heart of the sacred tree—to function properly, the spheres of Compassion and Judgment, which directly connect to it, must be kept in balance.

Beauty gets out of balance when you are constantly judgmental and rarely compassionate. If you are sabotaging Beauty then, on the physical level, you may be creating physical problems for yourself such as a hardening of the arteries.

Are you too willful or severe a person instead of one who practices loving kindness? Are there times when you replace justice with cruelty? Such attitudes miss the essence of spirit and can lead to ill health.

So if you want to prevent cardiac problems or are trying to recover from a heart condition, it is important that from now on you eliminate or reduce angry revengeful barbs.

Instead, practice values such as love and honor. Exercise patience and wisdom in all things. We act wisely when we fuse our human will and insight with cosmic intelligence and emerge as a flexible human being rather than a negatively willful one. This is the path to spiritual, physical, and emotional wholeness.

On the other hand, you might also ask yourself whether you have been too merciful over the years. It may seem like a strange question to ask, but according to Kabbalistic tradition, the role of Judgment is to curtail an overabundance of mercy, which can often degenerate into folly.

Have you been giving more than you can afford and receiving less than you should? That's one example of an overemphasis on mercy, which can lead to tension and health problems. Mercy is a wonderful trait, but only when reason is its companion.

If your answers to any of these questions fail to please you, that is a good sign. It means that you have conducted an honest appraisal of yourself and found that you lack a balanced attitude, which may be harming the energy center called Beauty.

Now is the perfect time to make a new start. Beginning and ending are activities of the same circuit. Whenever we begin again, something has to end. Whenever something has ended, it is because a new beginning has forced a change, just as a blade of grass forces a change in the earth so it can slip through.

So end your old ways and start anew. You don't need to change the world, only yourself. Concentrate on ridding yourself of any excessive or imbalanced behavior, whether it is being too judgmental, too passive, too enthusiastic, or whatever.

It is quite easy for Compassion and Judgment to become imbalanced. Here is a simple example. Let's say that I go out on the street right now and I happen to have one hundred dollars with me. I see a destitute homeless person, so I reach into my pocket and give him all my money. Then I go down to the subway and I don't even have enough cash to buy a ticket.

Was I a good and merciful man, or was my judgment way off?

Was I compassionate or foolish? I believe that I was a foolish man! I failed to combine compassion with good judgment. My thinking was not balanced.

Another way that Compassion and Judgment could have been thrown out of whack is if I had angrily said to this beggar: "Why don't you go out and work?" I then would have walked away feeling very annoyed with him. In this instance, my judgment overruled my compassion.

Imagine how Beauty would have reacted to such an outburst. She would have gone into hiding. And if I permitted this type of behavior to continue, the eventual result might be been a stroke or some other heart ailment.

Compassion and Judgment are extremes, which can only be harmonized by the sphere of Beauty. But this sphere requires nourishment to work her integral magic.

She is like a beautiful flower. If you fail to nourish her, she loses her luster and wilts. For good coronary health, you must pay attention to this sphere and the triad she is part of.

One excellent way to continually remind yourself of the importance of beauty and harmony involves the using of your hands. Let me explain. To drive a car we can use one hand. We can also use one hand to build something. We can even use one hand to physically attack someone. It's also possible to use one hand to embrace someone, although if anyone ever embraces you with one hand it really means they hate you!

But to remind us of beauty and harmony, when you arise in the morning use both hands to embrace the day. Make it a morning meditation. Use that gesture to symbolize that not only are you embracing this new day with confidence and enthusiasm, but also each moment of your life.

If you are reading this book while recovering from a heart ailment, an understanding of the various correspondences of this triad will help you keep heart-healthy.

Take a lesson from the world of economics. If, for example, you've had three bad years in business, and you're a little depressed, you might want to try meditating on what is going wrong at the office.

I guarantee that once you add intuitive skills such as meditation to your business acumen, you will do more business in the fourth year than all the previous three years combined.

The same holds true for your health problem. Do not become fixated by the old, worn-out patterns of behavior that may have led to your heart condition in the first place.

Instead, dare to begin again! Let the branches of the sacred tree unfold for you and enjoy the harvest of health this tree can offer you if you pay attention to her ways.

The more familiar you become with this magical tree, the more it will reveal to you its many secrets. You will then build a stronger heart the second time around.

The Third Triad:
Sexual and Gastrointestinal Problems

The third triad on the Tree of Life is comprised of Victory, Glory in Splendour, and Foundation. This triangle corresponds to the lower part of the body—the stomach and gastrointestinal tract, genitals, hips, loins, and legs. It is a cluster of spheres that represents the body and senses.

If you are having sexual or gastrointestinal problems, I suggest that you begin searching for the root of these health problems in this triad because something here is definitely out of balance.

Victory

Victory is about powerful desire, the sensuous quality of love, and how you view sex—whether you see yourself as a sexual conqueror or somebody who is more in God consciousness during the act of intercourse.

When meditating on Victory because of sexual problems—including impotence—you need to ask yourself honestly whether you have been excessively aggressive, boastful, or in other ways glorifying your ego in matters of sex.

If the answer to your question is "yes," then you should immediately begin to curb these baser instincts and excessive desires. You need to transmute them into a more pure and productive channel.

Remember what God asked Adam? "Where are you?" That is the primary question you need to ask yourself while meditating on this sphere (Victory). And if you don't like the reflection you see in your mental mirror, then seize the moment to meditate on Glory in Splendour and ask God for forgiveness: "I didn't realize what I was doing. I was excessive. I'm sorry." This can lead to healing.

Even in business, if your sole intent is conquest over a competitor at all costs, you need to let go of such an attitude as quickly as possible in order to maintain good health.

Such strong feelings may have caused you health problems already or will some day. Try tuning down such excessive behavior and, instead, practice a little humility.

Many gastrointestinal problems are caused by stress that comes from excessive behavior, such as trying too hard to be victorious in business or other areas of your life.

Conversely, if you remain too attached to the world of thoughts as represented by the sphere of Glory in Splendour, and are unable to take decisive action, you may become nervous and worried because of your inability to deal with obstacles and challenges.

This can also lead to stress and a host of gastrointestinal ailments. A little more Victory, or firmness, might be needed in your life to establish some balance between the two spheres.

Many gastrointestinal ailments are the result of poor diet and eating habits. Meditating on Victory and Glory will encourage you to think about your eating habits and any excesses connected to diet.

For example, are you eating animals because you believe that humans are superior to other creatures? This is a feeling associated with the sphere of Victory, which you need to work on.

Are you rushing through meals because closing a business deal is more important to you than proper digestion? This urge to create money rather than celebrating the sacred nature of the food you are eating is also an example of being in a Victory mode of thinking.

Powerful, uninhibited emotions identified with male potency can help destroy your body. You are placing too much value on triumph and achievement.

If all of this sounds familiar, try to tune down the ego a bit and see what happens to your digestive problems. Be hungry for a little more humility in the why and the way you eat.

Start thinking about honoring *all* life and about the sacred nature of food. I know that changing your eating habits can be very difficult. But you need not do it all at once. After all, even the spheres and the branches of the Tree of Life emanated one by one.

So change things regarding your eating habits one at a time. You don't have to eliminate all your bad habits all at once. By meditating on the spheres of Victory and Glory in Splendour, you will awaken to new ways of doing things. I predict that such changes will lead to physical improvement and create a future with no gastrointestinal problems.

Glory in Splendour

This sphere emphasizes the need to overcome your base emotions. It represents the more thoughtful side of uncontrolled instincts and emotions, and tries to purify carnal thoughts.

Meditating on Glory (thoughts) can certainly help put your life in perspective. It will serve to remind you to temper your strong instincts and emotions represented by Victory (feelings).

Glory also speaks of the importance of bringing loving thoughts of God into the act of procreation. But beware of placing too much emphasis on this sphere. That can throw you out of balance as well. If you are overly idealistic, too loving, and too accepting to the point of foolishness, the ultimate result will not be beneficial to your state of health.

One of the paths to freedom from illness and disease is through bringing Victory and Glory in Splendour into harmony. Then these two energies are able to strengthen the sphere of Beauty, as well as that of Foundation.

Foundation

Foundation gains its power through the union between Victory and Glory in Splendour. This sphere always strives to reflect Beauty, to which it is also connected.

This globe is the next to last stop on our journey downward through the Tree of Life. It leads directly to Kingdom, the tenth and final sphere through which we experience our world of the five senses. Foundation is one of your last opportunities to get your own Kingdom in order if you seek good health and healing.

When you meditate on Foundation think of the life you have created for yourself. Consider carefully whether you want to continue this type of lifestyle or, instead, work with God to build His/Her Kingdom on earth.

Because it is part of the triad of Victory and Glory in Splendour, Foundation also addresses the issue of humility versus pride. A showoff attitude; "I am a man/woman and I can conquer," or "I can have a new woman/man anytime I want," or "I can use every woman/man in any way I want," with an emphasis on Victory is a mistake. That sort of thinking does not build a solid foundation.

But again I caution you against too much humility, which can immobilize you and create an inability to overcome obstacles in your life. So when you meditate on Foundation, understand the need for balance between Victory and Glory in Splendour in order to remain grounded.

The sphere of Foundation is concerned with establishing a solid framework that you can build on. It is the framework for harmonious living, which is a vehicle for promoting good health.

If you feel that your foundation is still a shaky one, the following exercise, which is a meditation on Glory in Splendour, may be useful to you. First it requires that you perform a symbolic *mikvah*, which we discussed in chapter 6 (pages 77–78). Once you do so, then follow these steps:

Exercise

Visualize all the major organs of your body. All these organs are a part of you. Touch each part either physically or through visualization of your body, especially those parts that require healing.

Send the light of the Sabbath night candles or the light of candles from your own religious tradition to every organ of your body. Repeat the mantra or affirmation, "*The light of the Lord is the soul of man.*"

Hold up your ten fingers with palms towards you. Look at them and visualize the ten *sefiroth* of the Tree of Life or the Ten Commandments. See each of your fingers glowing with the light of God.

Next, place your fingers on the affected part or parts of your body. Then recite the words: *Neir Elohim.* It means "The light of God." Repeat these words at least ten times.

Now, in your mind's eye, visualize the sphere of Glory in Splendor.

See yourself in complete humility without pride. See yourself committed to creating for God—not your own ego—whether that creation is the conception of a child or the launching of some new business venture.

In this sacred moment, experience life's love for you, God's love for you, and your love of God. Feel faith, not fear. Calmness replaces agitation. A spiritual light now surrounds you. It shoots forth from the sphere of Glory in Splendour. You are in God's hands. You are healed.

End this meditation with gratefulness for your healing. Repeat the words, *"All is in divine order."*

Kingdom

The final sphere on the Tree of Life is The Kingdom, and it can be useful for healing. This is a very simple but extremely important globe. It represents the Kingdom of God on earth that we were put here to build. This sphere also corresponds to the entire body and its five senses.

The Kingdom is our home. It is planet Earth, the place where life began on the last day of creation. The Kingdom is the sum total of mind, body, and soul that we need to keep in harmony in order to do the Lord's work. It represents the best of us when we are feeling grounded and in harmony.

Meditate on this sphere to remind you of the Tree of Life healing work you have done either on yourself or someone else. It will also remind you that more healing work still needs to be done in partnership with God.

Although this sphere emphasizes the importance of the body and senses—of staying grounded—its direct connection to the Crown suggests that the health of the body cannot be maintained unless we also remain aware of our spiritual being.

One thing you might think about while meditating on The Kingdom is: "I'm healthy now or getting better. I'm beautiful. I have wisdom. I have knowledge. I have compassion and humility. What am I going to do with it?"

Hopefully, your answer will be, "I'm going to continue to build the Kingdom of God with God." This is exactly what you need to do to bring about an improvement in your health, because the final, ultimate mastery over your physical challenges will only come through union with the Lord.

So practice love and oneness; love and creation, not selfishness, which may have led to your disease in the first place. Remain aware that a feeling of spiritual oneness can lead to physical wholeness.

Get busy building that kingdom. Take action. Don't be like the man who has a million dollars and puts it under his mattress. Instead, do something with your money.

No matter what ailment you may have or how difficult your situation may be, know that you are now standing at The Kingdom, which is the Gate of the Garden of Eden. Revel in the knowledge that, having arrived at this gate, a new world of health and recovery will open for you.

My father was a gifted teacher, a rabbi who transformed those around him by his mere presence. He taught that all observable things here are reflected in a higher world, and that no person survives independently on any plane of existence, no matter how high that plane might be.

We've now been to that higher world and I hope that among the lessons you have learned is how interconnected we are with God and with each other, and just how important it is to keep that special relationship in proper order.

The universe and mankind share the same sea of harmony. The trick to sailing that sea is awareness that it is possible to do so. Anyone who is determined to heal or be healed, must listen to the inner voices of the spheres, which explain the proper way to sail the ocean of life.

In addition, you must also listen to the inner voices of God, the *Shekinah*, and your soul, which are filled with perennial wisdom and profound knowledge. These voices will always provide you with important keys to facing the challenges of your life and ill health.

Continue to keep your spiritual eyes open through this inward vision. Whenever necessary, return to the Tree of Life and taste its fruits. Affirm how sweet they are. Affirm "*it is good.*" Affirm that whatever health problems you may now be facing, nonetheless "*it is good to be alive!*"

Three Case Histories

"I have filled him with the spirit of God, with wisdom,
understanding, and knowledge."
—Exodus 31:2–3—

The great Jewish writer and healer, Maimonides, believed that when-ever one had an ailment in the body, it was simply a sign that there was something not right with the soul. I have come to that same con-clusion. We place ourselves in danger when we forget our purpose here on earth.

Kabbalah teaches that every person is unique and necessary, and that they must serve the Lord with joy, love, humility, and totality. Unfortu-nately, many of my clients seem to have forgotten that mission in life.

Instead, they are filled with painful problems, heartaches, anxieties, and the tragedies of life. They're like the driver of a car traveling down scenic Route 80 who finds an exit that says "McDonald's."

Pulling into McDonald's, the driver decides not to continue along life's beautiful road. He or she likes it here so much that they're going to stay. The driver forgets about his trip, about what he is supposed to do, and where he is supposed to be going.

That's what often happens when we get sick. We get sidetracked and fail to move on toward our goal of restoring balance to our body, mind, and soul. Instead, we can get very comfortable in a place that is not very healthy for us.

My role is to try to get the driver of the car back to Route 80 so that he or she can continue on their journey to health and happiness. For-tunately, I've been able to help some people find the road again, as the following three cases will show.

The first case involved a young woman who had what I immedi-ately sensed was a disease of the soul. This woman, who I will call Frieda, was someone who always complained about life rather than enjoyed it. I believe it was my Kabbalistic training rather than my skills as a therapist that was of most help to this unfortunate woman.

One day Frieda walked into my office and before she even sat down, she told me she felt as if she were dying. She was groaning, "Why me?" Then Frieda told me about all the physical things that were ailing her. She kept asking, "Why, why, why?"

Usually I don't stop anyone from talking. So when she finally finished, I looked at her and said, "Frieda, you know what your problem is? You're a *kvetch* (complainer)."

I went on to tell her that there was no answer to her "why" questions. I explained that it was like trying to answer the question of who created God? Or why we were born to suffer?

Instead, I offered her a Kabbalistic piece of advice. I suggested that from now on she focus on the question "How—How did I get all these problems? How can I still find joy?"

You see, there are two kinds of questions—bad questions and good questions. Bad questions have no answers, and good questions have thousands of answers. Who created God is a bad question. You can ask it from now to the end of your life and never get an answer.

But the good question is that if I accept the hypothesis that there is a God, what is it that God wants of me? For years this woman was asking the wrong question. She was totally lost. I decided that what she needed was what I call a "spiritual operation."

The spiritual operation I performed on her was a simple one. It involved me telling her: "You're a *kvetch* and this is not the real you. Where's your joy?" I was indirectly suggesting that she was exhibiting schizophrenic tendencies—that she was two people.

I said, "I'll tell you what you're going to do. You're going to bury that complaining personality. You're going to say *Kaddish* (the prayer for the dead) for that personality that you are burying." I told her to do this at midnight, and that ten minutes before midnight she should light a candle.

I advised Frieda to look at that candle and see herself the way she used to be, before she began complaining, crying, and feeling miserable about her life. I told her to see herself happy and healthy while standing in the light.

The next morning Frieda called and asked if she could see me.

When she walked into my office I didn't recognize her. She said, "I don't feel sick anymore. I feel like a new person." And she looked it. We both talked about it and we both cried about what had taken place.

What happened here demonstrated one of the most important Kabbalistic principles of all—the importance of making a soul-to-soul connection. As I listened to her, a connection was established between us and I said the right words.

For the first time in years, this young woman was able to see herself clearly. Reacting to my words, Frieda was able to make a decision right there and then that she didn't want to be that person I described—the *kvetch*. She didn't even want to be here in my office anymore, but back on that beautiful highway called life, and to life she returned. That healing came from God through me.

It had nothing to do with any psychoanalytic expertise. In the sacredness of that hour I was an extension of God. I was experiencing that intense moment called *Shutaf Elohim*, when we recognize with certainty that we are all partners with God.

During that first session I wasn't a husband, or a son, or a father, or a rabbi, or an analyst. I was nothing but an extension of my client. I had become one with her soul. That enabled me to sense her conflicting personalities and somehow make a connection to what was really causing her physical ailments. The result was healing.

Another case involved a wealthy fifty-year-old woman who came to me in physical and emotional distress. Irene was divorced, and her only interest now was her son.

She wasn't a very nice person. She was judgmental, full of anger, and I don't think she really ever loved her husband or her son. She needed them for her own selfish reasons.

Shortly before she came to see me, Irene and her son had an argument. Now they weren't on very good terms. On top of that, her son told her that he was in love with a woman on welfare who had three children. They planned to get married and live in a poor neighborhood on the city's upper west side. That was killing her! She had headaches, chest pains—everything! Irene was sick, sick, sick, and under a doctor's care. So the first thing I tried to apply was a little psychology.

I said to her, "My dear, the more you object to this marriage the deeper he will go into it, because it's a way of punishing you."

We talked about the situation. I asked Irene if the woman her son was in love with was the daughter of a king somewhere in Africa, would she still object to the marriage? "I don't know," she replied weakly.

So I immediately understood that it was not the fact that this woman was from a minority group, which galled her, but because she was poor. Next, I asked my client to concentrate on the spheres of Compassion and Judgment.

I told her to meditate on why it mattered to her that her son's girlfriend was poor. After all, maybe she was a beautiful human being? While meditating on the spheres, I had my patient imagine herself as being more compassionate and less judgmental.

This led to a discussion about humanity, and the Kabbalistic concept that we are all connected. Then I talked to her about the words from the sacred *Shemah Yisrael* prayer where it specifically states that we are all one—rich or poor, black or white, Protestant, Catholic, Hindu, Moslem, or Jewish.

After only three sessions we reached a point where Irene told me that she was at peace with the whole idea of her son's pending marriage. "It's his life," she declared. "Let him do what he wants." She had moved up to the sphere of Wisdom.

I felt that her whole attitude had changed because I introduced the spiritual idea that we are all one, and therefore should be in harmony with each other.

I had also assessed her energy centers according to the Tree of Life, and intuitively felt that Irene's illness was the result of an imbalance between the spheres of Compassion and Judgment.

She was a *Din*, or Judgment personality, and her lack of *Chesed*—Compassion—cut off her access to *Tifereth*, Beauty. The moment my patient let go of Judgment and focused her thoughts on Compassion, Irene not only felt better emotionally, but many of her physical symptoms—such as headaches—began to disappear.

I believe that the sphere of Judgment controls most of us most of the time. We are always being judgmental. Therefore it is advisable that we all meditate more on the sphere of Compassion if we want to remain healthy. This emphasis will transmute Judgment to justice. And where justice exists, then all is in divine order.

The last case I'd like to share with you involved a man who I will call Max. Max was a friend of a member of my congregation. He came to me for counseling after he had suffered a heart attack.

Max came to me feeling completely hopeless and in despair. He was angry at himself, his body, God—everybody. His medical report showed a complete blockage of the blood vessels to the heart.

I realized almost immediately that Max's body was not his enemy, but rather, his thoughts. Max was a businessman whose greatest joy seemed to be in winning his next deal.

Max approached his family and friends in a similar manner. He always liked to come out on top, whether in an argument with his wife or son, or his best friends. I could tell right away that Max was stuck in the sphere of Victory, and needed meditation work with the spheres of Splendor in Glory and Foundation.

His emphasis on the ego had blocked his access to the sphere of Beauty, which, as a result, impacted negatively on the spheres of Wisdom and Compassion.

In addition, I also discovered that Max ate a large amount of red meat. I suspected that all the red meat he consumed probably helped to fuel his aggressive behavior.

Max and I had a long road to travel before we could approach the subject of the Tree of Life. After all, how could he even begin climbing the healing tree when he was so out of shape on all his energy levels?

For several weeks we worked together on many different aspects of his lifestyle—from Max's diet to his obvious neglect of his spiritual life. We talked a lot about joy, and I finally managed to convince him to join a support group in order to deal with his feelings of anger and despair.

I tried to impress upon Max is that his heart attack was not something he needed to obsess about. Certainly that tragedy had caused him a lot of personal unhappiness, but I tried to explain that his anger was more of a hindrance than a help.

He needed to get through his compulsive thoughts and begin to co-create a new life with God. I quoted to him my favorite psalm (the twenty-third psalm) about "the valley of the shadow of death," and emphasized that the idea was to walk *through* that fearsome place, not linger the way he was doing.

During one session I described an ugly chair that I once had in my apartment. I told Max that I had learned to live around it, not sit in it. "Are you ready to do that?," I asked him.

"How do I get ready?" Max asked tentatively.

"Trust," I replied. "Find a new chair to sit in and have faith that you will feel very comfortable sitting there."

Eventually, we arrived at a point where Max was in a state of *hahanah*—readiness—not only to buy a new chair, but also to begin doing pathwork on the sacred tree.

To start our journey on the path of the sacred tree I asked Max to tell me a business story emphasizing Victory. I then retold the story from the perspective of Glory. During these storytelling sessions, we talked about his feelings when I offered my more spiritual version.

One afternoon, Max told me a story about a business deal in which he had bested his own brother. During the telling of this story, Max almost seemed to gloat that he had come out ahead in the transaction, although his brother could have used the extra money because he had a larger family.

In turn, I told this beautiful Talmudic story about genuine love:

There were two brothers who lived in the Holy Land. They were both farmers. They worked together and tilled the soil together. One brother was married and had a big family. The other brother was single.

Every year they would divide the harvest equally. One year, after they divided the harvest, the single brother said to himself, "Something is wrong here. I have taken exactly half of the harvest and I don't need that much. I have no wife or children. It's my brother who needs more."

So that night he couldn't sleep. In the middle of the night he got up, loaded his wagon, drove to the other side of the mountain where the younger brother lived, and left a portion of the harvest there.

The married brother couldn't sleep either. He said to himself, "Sure I have a family, and I need more. But when my brother gets old, who will take care of him? He needs protection for his old age. He really needs more than I. When my children grow up they can work and help their parents."

So he got up in the middle of the night, loaded his wagon, and drove to his older brother's house where he left a portion of the harvest there. The next morning when each brother got up, he found that he still had half of the harvest.

That night each of them loaded the wagon and left a part of the harvest at the other brother's house. And again, the third night, they did the same. They wondered what was happening.

Then on the fourth night, the brothers met right in the middle of the mountain. As they saw each other, they understood. They got off their wagons and embraced and kissed each other. According to Hassidic tradition, God observed their meeting and said, "This is the place where I want my temple built."

I don't know for sure what kind of impact my story had on Max, but by the middle of my story the smug smile on his face had vanished as the moral of the tale set in.

Gradually, Max began to get it. He began to see that Victory was not as important as gratitude, and that it was more important to identify with God than with the almighty dollar. Slowly but surely he came to see why his lack of balance may have led to his heart problem. That's when Max's healing really began.

Max now attends my Friday night Sabbath services and he is still working on his spiritual fitness program. I believe that his new awareness will help guard against a second, perhaps more fatal, heart attack.

It was through the lessons of the Tree of Life that Max learned an important spiritual truth: All we need to start a new way of living—one that will help ensure good health—is to trust in God's caring partnership with us.

Max continues to be a successful businessman, but he conducts business a bit differently now with a spiritual ally always at his side. He had faced his own self-destructive behavior and, as a result, inner peace was possible.

The Physician of the Soul

"In your name I lift my hands."
—Psalms 63: 5,7—

To be a Physician of the Soul, you must develop not only a loving attitude toward your fellow man, but to yourself as well. You also need to develop a trusting attitude toward God.

Whether your healing work is for yourself or others, you must approach it with a very definite commitment and a strong sense of awareness and dedication. Above all, always remain open to the possibility of miracles occurring in your life.

In your healing work, always listen to what your body or that of your client is trying to tell you with your "third ear," and "see" with your inner eye. As Physicians of the Soul, we are constantly called upon to listen and observe.

Sometimes when I listen, I "hear" the sound of a Mighty Presence speaking to me. I cannot pinpoint where the sound comes from. I know only that I must listen with my whole being to hear it.

I become so sensitive to this voice, like a Reiki master, even my fingers are filled with healing energy. Have you not heard the expression, "I am all ears?"

That expression has literal truth when we earnestly seek guidance. And if you seek to become a Physician of the Soul, you must also always be on the alert for the Divine Spirit who dwells in each one of us and guides us in our healing work.

When doing healing work on others, there are two cardinal rules you must always obey. First there must be a *soul to soul* connection. Only then can a healing can take place. You must feel that oneness between you, the client, and God.

Freud and Jung described this process as transference, and other psychotherapists over the years have given it all kinds of names. But the basic idea is that if you are doing healing work on someone with whom you don't feel comfortable, you better send that person to see someone else.

The second cardinal principle is that you must not attempt to heal someone without their permission. Furthermore, trying to heal someone who is not ready to receive your gift of healing in body, mind, and spirit, may have no effect whatsoever.

Spiritual Illnesses

As a Physician of the Soul, your main task will be to heal various spiritual illnesses, which can afflict us on our different energy levels.

While the Tree of Life is a powerful tool for the healing of such illnesses and bringing forth wholeness, there are some other spiritually based healing techniques that I would now like to share with you.

The Spiritual Injection

The first technique is one which I call "The Spiritual Injection." It is specifically designed to help heal a body that is spiritually ill. It can be used to help treat any part of the body that may be suffering discomfort.

You should put aside at least an hour for this healing work. Now turn the lights down for a few moments. You want to use your own inner light to guide you through this healing journey. Next, begin to meditate on the sphere or spheres of the Tree of Life that you believe are most related to the problem at hand.

If you are doing spiritual healing on someone else, you may allow your client to keep his or her eyes open until they close of their own accord. You are trying to guide them into the mystic trance state that was discussed in chapter 9.

Now, take your right hand, and with the thumb and forefinger form a circle. This circle represents *Ein Soph,* God, the Endless One, or infinity.

Through the use of this symbol, you are calling upon God and asking the Creator to send His/Her personal physician, the Archangel Rafael.

Creating this symbol is important for the healer. It signifies that

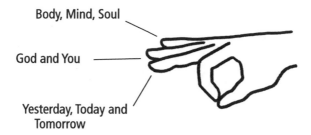

Body, Mind, Soul

God and You

Yesterday, Today and Tomorrow

Fig. 9: The Spiritual Injection

whatever healing work is being done is in the name of God with the help of this spiritual messenger.

The three remaining fingers of the right hand are also powerful symbols. From right to left, they stand for the triad of Crown, Wisdom, and Knowledge. They also signify God's name as it is known in the Kabbalah—*Shin*—whose Hebrew letters are a shortcut version of the word "*Shekinah.*"

Now look at your right hand. Visualize it as a powerful tool for healing. The high priests of ancient Israel used various hand gestures when they approached the Holy of Holies, which was a sacred room in the temple bare of everything but the spirit and glory of God. So sanctify your hand as a symbol of sanctifying God. Say out loud, "I have God in my hands."

Sometimes I ask my clients to make a meditation out of this blessing. Often, I join them in repeating those words. If you are doing healing work on yourself, meditate on this blessing for a few moments.

Now take the three fingers and begin the "spiritual injection." Touch the area of discomfort in a rolling motion with the middle finger first, ring finger second, and the pinkie last.

The middle finger represents "yesterday, today, and tomorrow," the ring finger symbolizes "God and you"—*the Shekinah*—and the pinkie represents "body, mind, and soul."

Next, reverse this process. Gently apply the "Spiritual Injection" with the three fingers beginning from right to left, starting with the

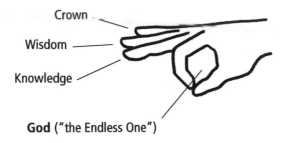

Crown

Wisdom

Knowledge

God ("the Endless One")

Fig. 10: The Spiritual Injection

pinkie. Now, with all three fingers together in one motion, touch the area of the body that you are working on. Repeat this "injection" seven times. The number seven in the Kabbalah represents the seven heavens.

Meditate on these seven heavens. See the angels going up and down between the heavens. Feel the healing power in your fingers growing stronger. Also meditate on the will to live and the need to have compassion for yourself and others. Repeat the affirmation, "*I want to live.*"

If you are doing healing work on someone else, quietly explain what you are doing throughout this technique. This subdued conversation will help to induce a mystical trance. You want that person to close their eyes and relax.

Suggest to them (or to yourself) that any pain or discomfort, which they may be experiencing, is vanishing as they hear these words. Ask them to meditate on whatever sphere or spheres you are incorporating into your healing.

Now repeat out loud the following affirmation: "*I want to live.*" This is a very important affirmation, and one which I use regularly in my own daily meditation practice.

The second part of this healing technique is applicable to all parts of the body. If, for example, the pain you are trying to eliminate is in the head area, take your three fingers and touch the forehead.

Next, with all five fingers of your hand held close together, make a circular sweep over the forehead three times. Follow this with the same sweeping motion over the back of the head.

Now make this circular hand gesture over the right ear—Knowledge—and then the left ear—Wisdom. If the healing work was centered on the lower part of the body, then these sweeps would be made first on the left side of the body—Glory in Splendour—followed by the right side—Victory.

Let's return to our example of the head. With your whole right hand and fingers spread wide apart, make a wide circular motion around the face. Repeat this seven times. What you are doing now is cleansing the aura, that spiritual energy field which surrounds all living beings.

By cleansing the aura, you not only get rid of all the negativity that may have contributed to the disease, but you are replacing it with a new awareness—a new kind of thinking—that is more positive.

The "Spiritual Injection" technique is now complete. Repeat out loud: "All is in Divine Order." This may be an excellent moment for some silent prayer. Visualize health being restored to your body or the person you are working on. Thank God and the Archangel Rafael for their assistance in your healing.

Chanting the Holy Name

Often, when I perform the "Spiritual Injection" during my healing work, I chant out loud one of the sacred names of God (see Chapter Eight). I do this whenever I feel the spirit to do so. It's a spontaneous moment.

The Holy Name I prefer to chant is *Shadai*, which contains within in the root of the Hebrew word *dayanu*, meaning enough. *Dayanu* also suggests that God is filled with compassion. Even if there is pain and suffering, it doesn't necessarily mean that things won't change. There's no reason to stop believing in the sun even when it doesn't shine.

Amazing results are produced when people who are ill learn that there is a positive message of health, healing, and hope in the name of God that I chant.

So many of us have become accustomed to the concept of eternal suffering. Even the Christian concept of Jesus reinforces this way of thinking—we did something wrong so He had to *suffer* and die for our sins.

Some people who come to me for healing interpret their illness or pain as "It's coming to me, I must have done something wrong." They usually believe that their disease is a permanent punishment from God.

In my home as a child, whenever something went wrong I would hear my mother say, "It is God's punishment." Although I know differently now, I still remember that easy answer to life's difficulties. I no longer believe that when something bad happens to us it is "God's will." Neither do I believe that God intends for us to suffer permanently. I certainly recognize that bad things can happen to good people, but I also pay close attention to the fact that God's name contains the positive message—"enough! enough already!"

While I agree that it is sometimes very difficult to reconcile the concept of a God of love and a universe infused with a loving spirit with the worldly experience of suffering, my personal approach is to try and remain joyous even in the face of adversity.

I try to explain to those I counsel that it is not necessarily God who is responsible for their physical or emotional problems. Rather, they may have allowed themselves to get into a state of disharmony on certain energy levels.

I also try to make the point that God does not punish us by separating Himself/Herself from us. Any separation from God occurs when you or I choose the separation. God does not choose to be separate from us. Keep that thought in mind and I promise that you'll never feel alone.

Do not feel sad or melancholic. I have certainly experienced the cruelty and hardness of the world, beginning with the Nazi holocaust in which I lost most of my family. I still remember that God said, "*Ki Tov*"– *it is good!* I call this "God's mantra," and I repeat it often to myself. I distinguish between happiness and joy. And although I often am not happy, I am always joyous.

Another Holy Name I use when I chant during the "Spiritual Injection" is *El Melach Ne-emon.* This means "God the King in whom I trust." You have to put your life and your sickness in the hands of God who is sending his angel, Rafael, to heal you.

Sometimes I simply meditate on that name and, at other times, I follow that silent meditation with the chanting of the Holy Name. It really doesn't matter if you chant God's holy names in Hebrew or in any other language. His/Her name invoked in Sanskrit or English is just as powerful as the Hebrew version. I repeat my invocations in Hebrew because I feel a connection to that language. I can hear my forefathers four thousand years ago chanting the same prayers in the same language. I visualize the ancient Hebrew priests standing before the Holy of Holies waiting for word from God that all is in divine order. There is great power in that connection. It makes me feel that I'm not a leaf by myself, but part of that big tree. And I try to pass that feeling on to those to whom I am giving a spiritual healing.

The Power of an Embrace

There are moments when you are doing healing work—whether for yourself or others—that an embrace becomes very important. When you embrace another person—or even when you wrap your arms around yourself—you are creating a circular motion that represents your partnership with God. That's why you are and why you are here. You need God and He/She needs you. This gesture symbolizes the oneness of spirit.

I recall a man who came to me for spiritual healing, and toward the end of our session one of the most remarkable things happened! I don't know how the thought came to me – it was almost as if I were acting as a channel for the Almighty – but I decided to embrace him.

This feeling of being acted upon by some spiritual power frequently happens to me. At those moments, I am directed to express the will of God; I become a vessel of the Divine.

This was one of those moments. Until then, Richard barely spoke and, when he did, it was in such a subdued voice that I could hardly hear him. Suddenly, something told me, "embrace him!" Well, I wrapped my arms around this man and he almost fell apart with joy.

I think this was the first time in his life that anyone ever embraced him with a heart full of love and compassion. He completely opened up. Richard came to me a few more times and he was an entirely different person.

To me, that experience was an affirmation of how important touch is. I teach all my Kabbalah students about the need to embrace each other. This is also another example of what I mean by "soul to soul" contact. Of all the elements that are involved in spiritual healing, none is as important as a soul to soul encounter—embracing each other.

True Healing

True healing is not only about helping people in this lifetime, but also preparing them for the next one as well. A true healing will help correct what was done wrong in this lifetime, so that the next lifetime can be entered with a clear spirit.

In the Hindu tradition, it is believed that whatever your last thoughts are—good, positive, or negative—that is how you are going to begin your next life.

When Gandhi was assassinated, his last words to his assassin were, "I forgive you." Gandhi was healing his own soul of anger. He didn't want to begin his next life with anger, but with forgiveness.

So if you are doing healing work with a person who is dying, remember you are not healing the person in this life, but helping him or her to prepare their soul for the next. You can't really do anything more for a dying person in this lifetime. But if that person has any guilt or unresolved problems, then you need to try to heal him or her of those feelings.

Finally, to be a Physician of the Soul—to be an effective healer—the basic Kabbalistic principle to remember is to trust in God. If you don't have that faith, your healing will fail. Always remember that as a healer you are the ambassador of the Lord.

Always visualize the person with whom you are working (or yourself) as a Tree of Life. And don't worry about cures, because if the healing is done correctly, the cure will occur automatically.

The Spiritually Ill Soul

Like Maimonides, I believe that all sickness in the body originates in the soul. When the soul becomes ill, some physical or mental ailment usually accompanies it. Some symptoms of a spiritually ill soul are feelings of worthlessness, alienation, and hatred.

A soul that needs healing is always sending out S.O.S. (Save Our Soul) signals. But unlike the mind and body, the soul sends us her signals very quietly. Unless you have learned the art of listening, you may miss those signals.

Sometimes the soul says, "the only way I can get this person's attention is by doing something with the body that they can feel." If there is no other way for the soul to get your attention, you may develop a headache, eye trouble—all kinds of things. It's your wake-up call from the soul.

Flaw of the Saints

Sometimes, however, you may offend the soul in a way that it is difficult for you to understand. You may believe you have done nothing wrong. This is what I call the "flaw of the saints." It's not that you did something terribly wrong, you simply didn't realize—you weren't aware— that you did anything wrong.

When the Israelites were wandering in the desert and in desperate need of water, Moses, eager to help his thirsty people, struck a rock. He wasn't aware at the time that by so forcefully striking the rock he was harming one of God's creatures. God punished him by not allowing Moses to enter the Holy Land. Moses' action is an example of a saintly flaw.

Another saintly flaw is not actually performing an action that is wrong, but thinking about it. This is also an insult to the soul.

For example, a mother is angry at her child. She loves the child, but she may say, when the child misbehaves, "I'll kill you if you do that again." That's a version of a saintly flaw. She would never kill her child, but by saying such a thing, she was subconsciously thinking about bringing harm to her child, and wasn't even aware of it.

As a Physician of the Soul, you will often be called upon to heal a spiritually ill soul. You can bring about a healing through meditation, by listening to the soul's silent language—paying attention to and gaining guidance from that still small voice.

If you are doing healing work on another person, you must also awaken that person to the idea of listening to his or her soul. They must become aware that the soul exists to remind us each day of our lives that we're here for a purpose.

Our existence here is not an accident. Your birth may not have been planned, but was the result of two people sleeping together. But once you are born there is a real purpose to your life, and that purpose is to become one with God.

I think more medical doctors should become Physicians of the Soul and learn the art of spiritual healing. They need to become aware, as you are now, that many of our body's ailments are connected to problems of the soul.

Even I sometimes need such a reminder. Which makes me recall an incident that took place just the other day. This little boy, who is a member of my congregation, saw my hearing aid. He said, "Rabbi, my grandmother has something like that."

I looked at him and said, "My hearing aid is different. I can hear you and I don't really need it. I need it to hear God." And in a way, it's true. My hearing aid serves to remind me that God is always talking to us via our souls, and that many physical ailments which we suffer are the result of failing to listen to that voice.

Nightmares

Bad dreams or nightmares are also warnings from the soul that it is in need of attention. As a Physician of the Soul you need to pay close attention and carefully analyze any nightmare you or your client has had.

Ask yourself, "Why am I having these dreams? Does it have to do with something I've done or was going to do?" Whenever you or a client has a nightmare, you know that the soul has somehow become disconnected.

It's much like my telephone, which is a very unusual phone. When I stop talking or you stop talking it turns itself off. Interpreted spiritually, the phone is telling me that if I'm not talking to you and you're not talking to me, then we're disconnected. It's the same thing the soul is trying to tell you if you are having nightmares. That you have somehow become spiritually disconnected.

If you or someone you are trying to heal is experiencing nightmares, do not worry about it, but find out why this is happening. You may want to do meditation work or, if that fails to provide you with an answer, seek spiritual counseling from a more experienced Physician of the Soul.

Worthlessness and Alienation

These are among two of the most common afflictions of the soul. Worthlessness and alienation affect many people who come for spiritual healing.

How can anyone who is aware of the *Shekinah*, the Goddess within, suffer from feelings of worthlessness and alienation? You are not a failure. You're in partnership with God and that's got to be worth more than a million dollars. To feel worthless is an insult to the God within you.

Every man is a prince and every woman is a princess, and God is a king. All of us are His/Her sons/daughters. We're all children of God, so we're all princes and princesses.

As a prince I have things to do to keep my kingdom in harmony. I have a tremendous responsibility, which leaves me no time to dwell on thoughts like worthlessness.

If you stay in God consciousness through awareness, meditation, and prayer, you are somebody—a prince or princess. It should never even occur to you that you're worthless or alienated or that you're nothing.

Feelings of worthlessness and alienation are not a sickness. They are symptoms of a spiritually ill soul, and you can do something about it. All you need to do is increase your awareness of who you are and what God wants you to do in building His kingdom on earth.

The Letter Shin

In the Kabbalistic tradition, there is a central idea that each of us is a Tree of Life. There is also another concept that each of us is the *Shin* (see Fig. 1, page 30), the twenty-first letter of the Hebrew alphabet.

This is a very sacred letter. It stands for *Shekinah*, the in-dwelling God, and it also stands for *Shadai*, one of God's sacred names. This *shin* also stands for *shalom*, meaning peace.

In my efforts to heal spiritually ill souls, I make a living meditation out of that letter. I lift both my arms over my head, and the trunk of my body completes the third, or middle, stem of S*hin*.

This letter can represent different things according to where it is punctuated for emphasis. If the dot, which punctuates this letter, is placed to the right, (see Fig. 11B), then you have *Shin*. If the dot is to the left, we have, instead, "sin" (see Fig. 11A). The punctuation point makes all the difference between *Shekinah, shalom,* and sin.

During a healing session, I sometimes have my client meditate on the punctuation point to see where the dot is in his or her life. I also have them meditate on the middle stem of this three-pronged letter, which is the balance point between the two outer stems.

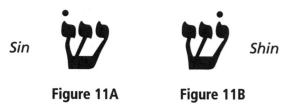

Sin　　　　　　　　　　　　　　　*Shin*

Figure 11A　　　　　**Figure 11B**

Sometimes as a joke I will say to my Kabbalah students, "The question is not what is your sign, but where is your dot?" This dot is also found in the first letter of the first Hebrew word of the Bible—*Bereshet,* meaning in the beginning.

If you remain aware of this *Shin,* and combine it with a meditation on the first triad of the Tree of Life, you will be taking major steps to eliminate any feelings of worthlessness and alienation. You will become the *shin.*

I am the shin. My mind has become mindful as the Buddha. My eyes now see the good in everything and everybody.

My ears are trained to listen for the good tidings of the coming of the Messiah and refuses to be tempted by pessimism or despair. My mouth is trained to observe the noble silence that the Buddhists talk about and, at the same time, also to know when to speak up for justice and righteousness.

My hands are trained to embrace all of God's children and all of life. My heart is trained to be compassionate and understanding. My feet are trained to run whenever I can be of help to somebody. All of this is who I am because the dot is now on the right side of my shin.

A Dying Choice

Sometimes I'm asked, "Suppose you're dying. What choices do you have here?" I reply, " 'You can choose to die angry or at peace with yourself."

Wouldn't you rather choose to die with the kiss of God on your lips like Moses did?

I'm sure Moses was feeling frustrated—even worthless—because he so much wanted to enter the land of Israel that God promised him and his people. Were all his efforts so meaningless that he wasn't allowed to step foot onto the Promised Land?

But instead of anger Moses chose joy. He said, "All right, God told me I couldn't enter the land of Israel. But let me rejoice in the fact that my children are going to enter that land."

Practice Joy

We've talked a lot about the importance of joy throughout this book. It's also important to mention joy as it applies to the healing of the spiritually ill soul. Lack of joy is definitely an illness of the soul.

If you are handicapped as a result of some disease—perhaps you are confined to a wheelchair and can no longer walk—then instead of concentrating on the fact that you cannot walk, watch people who can walk and rejoice in the fact that they are able to do so. That's one way to try and promote joy in your life.

I say this from personal experience. I have problems with my legs. I can walk, but I cannot run. I used to sit in Central Park near my house and envy all the joggers. But eventually I came to rejoice in their ability to run, and, as a result, I felt much better about myself and life than I did when I was feeling envious.

If you can learn to practice this kind of joy, you have attained the highest form of spirituality. Try for an attitude of "if I can't do it, if I can't have it, then let me rejoice in the fact that somebody else can." That is giving. That is love and optimism. These are thoughts that can certainly help heal the spiritually ill soul.

Hatred

Hatred is another disease of the soul. To me hatred is a poison just like anger is. And do you really want to poison yourself? We believe that if we hate someone we are hurting them, but the only one we are really hurting is ourselves. We are poisoning our own souls and will eventually suffer the consequences, perhaps as some kind of physical ailment.

As a Physician of the Soul, in order to promote health and healing, you must try to transcend the atmosphere of darkness that clouds the sphere of Beauty. You must replace hatred with love. If someone hates you, that's their problem. Don't hate them in return. Instead, be available to share your love, to give it to yourself or to people who need you. That's your responsibility. But you are not responsible for sharing the hatred someone may express toward you by returning that negative emotion.

We have six organs with which to serve God, but we are masters of only three of them. We cannot control our eyes, ears, and noses. But we can control our mouths, hands, and feet. So let's speak only words of kindness, do acts of charity, and get involved in noble causes.

Hatred can cause much illness—from high blood pressure to heart disease. Is that worth hating someone for? Why would anyone want to hurt themselves spiritually or physically with such a negative attitude? You only end up paying twice.

Letting Go

To heal a soul full of hatred, you must learn to let go. Meditating on the sphere of Compassion is one way to do so. To let go is to flow with the cosmic tide of rhythm and balance and to remove the personal self, with its companions of fear and futility, from the universal aura, which is always positive.

When I am counseling clients who are consumed with hatred—they hate their husbands or their wives or their kids or their employers and so on—in addition to suggesting that they meditate on the sphere of Compassion, I talk to them about the importance of cultivating inner peace.

Peace is a spiritual action. It is not a static, placid existence without challenges. It is an awareness that maximum peace comes from a mature ability to cope with hatred, anger, and frustration in a mature way.

Toward this end, I ask my clients to meditate on the sphere of Wisdom as well. Peace comes with wisdom, which we foster as we explore, evaluate, adjust, and adapt to people, problems, and ourselves.

So let hatred go! Believe me, it's easier than resisting. It only takes a change in point of view and the sails are set for forward movement.

The Kingdom of God

In order to heal a spiritually ill soul, meditate not only on Beauty, but also on all ten attributes of God on the Tree of Life as well—especially The Kingdom.

Always include the sphere of The Kingdom in such a meditation, because your basic goal in life is to build the Kingdom of God on earth. And that cannot be accomplished with hatred in your heart.

Meditation is always an excellent way to help heal sicknesses that affect the soul. In a meditative state you are likely to hear *Ruach Hakodesh,* the actual source of the soul's voice.

The *Ruach Hakodesh* can be compared to the source of transmission when you turn on your radio or television set. It is "the place" of the Holy spirit, the origin of your soul.

When I do soul healing work on myself of others, one prayer I'm fond of using is: *O God, the Soul that Thou has given me is pure. It is my job to keep it pure.*

The Spiritually Ill Mind

Why does the mind become spiritually ill in the first place? That's a hard question to answer. Let me share with you my own non-scientific theory that resulted from a personal tragedy that I suffered more than twenty-five years ago.

I was then married to my wife who developed Alzheimer's Disease. She was a very beautiful and highly educated person. She was a social worker and the director of the Grand Street Settlement House in New York City.

This very wonderful and active woman had all the positive aspects of the Tree of Life. And then, toward the end, her mind was affected to the point that she didn't even recognize me. I was sometimes her father and sometimes her son.

I'm not a doctor, so the reason I formulated for her affliction did not result from a study of medicine. I believe her disease came about as a result of jealousy, which is a spiritual illness of the mind. It began when the board of directors of the Grand Street Settlement wanted to be nice to her, so they hired a twenty-five-year-old assistant.

I think it was then that her mind went into crisis. She became distraught and felt that at age sixty she was no longer useful. Although the board members told her that she was working too hard and they wanted to get her some additional help, she didn't believe them.

Whatever her new assistant did she took the wrong way. She thought he was plotting against her. I suggested to my wife that if she felt so distraught about the situation, she should resign and rejoice in the fact that she had been of so much service to the agency over the years.

But no! Her jealousy grew, and I think that affected her mind. She had become spiritually ill and was trying to destroy herself and destroy everything that she had built with the agency over the years.

I learned many painful lessons from that experience. Today, when I deal with clients who suffer with problems like jealousy or anxiety, I try to emphasize that we need to train our minds not to respond to such strong emotions. I suggest to them that their sphere of Victory is out of balance.

If we are all one with God and the universe, then there is no room for jealousy, hatred, or whatever. That is how I trained my own mind when it came to the joggers I used to watch in the park. Instead of being jealous or envious because I was unable to run, I rejoiced in their ability to do so.

If you can train yourself to be joyous, then you are keeping your emotions spiritually healthy and your mind psychologically sound. I believe you are also acting to help keep your mind from being affected by some kind of physical illness such as Alzheimer's.

When we go see a movie or a play, we don't envy the characters on the screen or on stage who are able to do things that we can't do. Instead, we enjoy them.

If we can train ourselves to feel that way, and eliminate feelings like jealousy, envy, greed, and replace these feelings with "I don't have it, but they have it, and isn't that wonderful," then we are promoting good mental health.

Anxiety and Worry

Many of my clients come to me with problems related to anxiety. They're worried about this thing or that thing. Worry and anxiety are spiritual illnesses of the mind.

If my patients are worried and are trying to do something about their anxiety, that's great! But plain worrying without any action isn't going too resolve anything.

I recently had a client who told me that her mother was very sick and she was worried about it. I told this woman the story of the jeweler.

A young lady sees a beautiful ring in the window of the jewelry store. She goes into the store and asks the shopkeeper, "How much is it?" The jeweler says that the ring costs $10,000. The woman says, "Oh, it's beautiful but I can't afford it."

This woman was practicing "good" emotions. She felt a positive emotion toward the ring – she loved it – but was sensible enough not to allow her inability to purchase the ring to cause her anxiety, stress, or worry. She simply let it go!

The same holds true if your mother or some other person you are close to becomes ill. If that person needs you constantly, you can't afford being there all the time for the sake of your own mental health.

I always ask myself, "If I worry, will that help others?" The answer, of course, is no! Worry can only destroy you, so you have to stop worrying. Worry and agitation are a bottleneck.

These emotions are a hindrance and a deterrent to right action. What results is not love, but, more often, hostility and failure. It sets off a cycle of guilt and frustration.

If you are a worrier, think instead about enjoying this day. Worry, or a sense of doom, is one way we try to relieve the pressure of facing our own inertia in conquering the challenges of our environment.

It is an escape door to avoid constructive, courageous, imaginative action. It is a sellout, a betrayal of the zest of living! So focus on positive thoughts. This is one way you can try to retrain your mind. If you don't, worry is another poison that can result in poor health.

Visualization is an excellent way to help retrain the mind. The following exercise will help you when you are worried or anxious.

Exercise

Get comfortable, and breathe deeply. You may wish to use the breathing exercise described in chapter 3. Now visualize yourself and God walking through the Garden of Eden.

God is saying, "Let there be light." You look around and see this wondrous light shining on all the lush vegetation that grows in the garden. Repeat to yourself several times, "How enjoyable. What a beautiful walk God and I are taking together. We're actually walking through the Garden of Eden."

You are now in a state of mind where you have no worries. You have no anxieties. You're feeling safe and happy with God as your companion. You're now making a friend of your worrying mind.

Speak to your mind. Repeat several times: "Come on mind, come on mind, join me in this beautiful walk." This is a form of self-hypnosis that will help lead you to a deep level of meditation and ease your anxiety.

There is another quick and easy-to-do technique which I practice each morning. I look at myself in the mirror, and I say to myself, "Come on, Joseph, who are you really?"

I peer at my reflection and I laugh at myself. It helps to shake off my worries and anxieties. That's the lighthearted state of mind I want to be in before I begin my meditation.

This simple technique is based on an important Kabbalistic concept. When you look at your reflection, and laugh, you are stepping away from your own self-image, so that you can become aware that you are really a "He/She" instead of an "I."

You recognize that a spiritual power resides in you, and promises to share its power. That's an excellent way to emancipate yourself from anxiety and worry.

Health cannot be maintained or regained if you are a slave to emotions such as worry. Instead, you must try to free yourself from such mental turmoil and concentrate on developing your spiritual powers and your connection to the Almighty.

When you begin to feel that you are getting caught in worry's grasp, try repeating this affirmation: "*There is no problem, however difficult, that God and I together cannot handle.*" This kind of thinking is the way to self-liberation from the mental tyrants of anxiety and worry.

I have often thought it would be helpful to have a little Tree of Life that you could hold in your hands. I'd give them to all my clients who are suffering from a spiritually ill body, soul, or mind, so that they can be reminded that they are Trees of Life. I would have inscribed on that miniature Tree of Life a saying attributed to a wise Hassid—Rabbi Shlomo of Karlin—who once said: "The greatest evil is to forget that you are the child of a King."

So when anxiety and worry have you in their grasp, say to yourself: "*I am the son of a King. I don't have time for anxiety and worry. I have things to do here to help establish God's kingdom on earth and I'm going to do them.*"

Closing Thoughts

There is a story about the Baal Shem Tov that is still told throughout the world today. The Jews living in a community in Russia or Poland were afraid of a pogrom, a campaign of "ethnic cleansing." They went to the Baal Shem Tov for help. They said, "Pray for us, we are in great danger. They want to kill us all."

The Baal Shem Tov went into the forest, kindled a light, and said a special prayer. A miracle took place, and the community was saved. Even as this was happening, however, the Baal Shem Tov reminded the community that a time would come when he would no longer be there. They would have to learn to help themselves.

They helped themselves with the simplest tool they knew—singing. Sung in private or together with others, a simple melody has enormous power to bring peace of mind. When you are praising God in melody, you are joyous and at peace. Negative thoughts cannot enter your mind.

So learn to sing, my friends, or at least learn to dance!

Our quest in this book has been a search for reunion with our potential for good health and healing. This quest includes steering clear of despair, and transforming thoughts that distract you from the love of God into a joy of life. This is how inner wholeness and health is best attained.

Always remember that life resembles a tree. A tree has both straight and crooked branches. The symmetry of the tree, however, is perfect. Life is balanced like a tree.

It is beautiful and perfect despite the struggles, difficulties, and sorrows that are part of it. So taste the Tree of Life, my friends. Dare to taste the Tree and affirm it. *It's good to be alive. I am happy and joyous to be alive.*

This knowledge will hasten the coming of the Messiah and bring you good health as well.

God loves you. *Shalom*, my friends, *shalom....*

Healing Prayers

I often recite these prayers with clients who request spiritual healing. Use them like arms that can embrace with warmth. Let them bring life and health into their fullest bloom in your life.

Remember to pray with feeling and with the confidence of knowing that all the perfection that exists within the Higher Power is already present within you as a gift of love. Let these prayers instill in you peace of mind, and carry with them not only God's blessings, but my own as well.

1.

My soul aches to receive your love
Only by the tenderness of your light can she be healed.
Engage my soul that she may taste your ecstasy.

My heart yearns with an age-long yearning for the embrace of
  your compassion.
O God, penetrate my longing with your presence.

Hurry, my loved one. Embrace me that I may rejoice in the
  source of all joy.

2.

You are my Light and my Salvation
  whom shall I fear?
When I am filled with sorrow you soothe my soul.
You are the source of my strength and my comfort.

O God, comfort me now, fill me with your love in the morning,
  that I may sing joyously throughout the day. Balance my suf
  fering with joy.

Show me your wonders and loving care.
Be gracious to me, O God.

3.

God, help me to open my heart to you. Accept my prayers.
I thank you for the many joys you have given me.
For family and for friends,
    for the miracles of nature,
    the wonder of morning and the comfort of night.
For the peace of this day and the hope of redemption.
Thank you for your wisdom and the gift of Life.
Help me O God to find peace in myself and among all people.

4.

O my God—
This is the day the Lord created to be joyous and content.

I am the candle lit by a spark from God.
Toward the heavens my bright flame reaches adding light to the
    world around me.

5.

Adonai Elohim, O God
    keep my tongue from evil and my lips from speaking guile.

Be my support when grief silences my voice, and my comfort
    when woe bends my spirit.

Implant humility in my soul, and strengthen my heart with
    perfect faith in Thee.

Help me to be strong in temptation and trial and to be patient
    and forgiving when others wrong me.

Guide me by the light of Thy counsel, that I may ever find
    strength in Thee, my Rock and my Redeemer. Amen.

6.

(From Psalm 6)
…Be gracious to me Adonai
for I am desolate…
Heal me Adonai…
Heal and free my soul Adonai
Deliver me for the sake of your loving kindness.
Depart from me all evil doers
You must have heard my weeping.
Adonai has heard my supplication
Adonai will also accept my prayers.

Glossary

Baal Shem Tov. Rabbi who founded the mystical Hassidic sect in eighteenth century.

Binah. Sphere on Tree of Life representing knowledge.

Chesed. Sphere on Tree of Life representing compassion.

Chokhmah. Sphere on Tree of Life representing wisdom.

Devekut. Cleaving to God or being conscious of the Oneness of the Lord.

Din. Sphere on Tree of life representing judgment.

Etz Hayim. Tree of Life.

Gematria. Kabbalistic system for manipulating numbers to gain secret knowledge.

Hakol Baseder. Hebrew expression for "all is in divine order."

Hassidism. Eighteenth century Jewish mystical sect.

Hahanah. A state of readiness.

Hozeh. Vision.

Kabbalah. Hebrew word meaning to receive or reveal.

Kavanah. An awareness of God.

Kether. Sphere on Tree of Life representing the crown, or divine infusion.

Ki Tov. Hebrew expression meaning "praise life" or "all is good."

Lo amut. Hebrew expression meaning, "I shall not die."

Malkut. Sphere on Tree of Life representing the Kingdom of God on earth.

Modeh Ani. Morning prayer praising God for returning one's soul.

Mogen David. Star of David or Shield of David.

Nefesh. Lowest level of the soul.

Neshama. Soul.

Netzach. Sphere on Tree of life representing victory or pride.

Rafael. Archangel of healing.

Ruach. Highest level of the soul.

Sefiroth. Spheres or globes which represent various manifestations of God.

Sepher Yetzereth. Kabbalistic text supposedly written in the second century A.D.

Shekinah. Feminine aspect of the Divine.

Shemah. Best-known Hebrew prayer, repeated five times daily.

Shutaf Elohim. Hebrew expression meaning "partnership with God."

Tifereth. Sphere on Tree of Life representing beauty.

Torah. First five books of the Old Testament.

Yehovah. Hebrew word for God.

Yesod. Sphere on Tree of Life representing the foundation.

Yetzer harah. Bad inclination or impulse.

Yetzer hatov. Good inclination or impulse.

Zohar. Kabbalistic text supposedly written in thirteenth century Spain.

BOOKS BY THE CROSSING PRESS

Changing the World One Relationship at a Time: Focused listening for Mutual Support and Empowerment
By Sheryl Karas

Could you use some support so that you can go after the life of your dreams? *Changing the World One Relationship at a Time* will provide you with the information, skills, and practice you need to arrive at a more joyous life.

$10.95 • Paper • ISBN 0-89594-945-8

Clear Mind, Open Heart:
Healing Yourself, Your Relationships and the Planet
By Eddie and Debbie Shapiro

The Shapiros offer an uplifting, inspiring, and deeply sensitive approach to healing through spiritual awareness. Includes practical exercises and techniques to help us all in making our own journey.

$16.95 • Paper • ISBN 0-89594-917-2

Complete Guide to Tarot
By Cassandra Eason

Cassandra Eason makes a popular form of divination accessible and inviting, even for beginners and skeptics. She gradually builds to advanced topics, including cleansing a deck, keeping a tarot journal, analyzing complex spreads, and incorporating tarot into practices like the Kabbalah and numerology.

$18.95 • Paper • ISBN 1-58091-068-8

Conscious Marriage: From Chemistry to Communication
By John C. Lucas, Ph.D.

What are the tools of effective relating? Why don't we utilize them as we should in relationships? What has caused the cycle of dysfunction that has typified so many marriages in the past few decades? How do we grow beyond it? Lucas provides answers to these questions with a blueprint for building a successful relationship.

$14.95 • Paper • ISBN 0-89594-915-6

Dreams and Visions: Language of the Spirit
By Margaret M. Bowater

Dreams and Visions is an easy-to-follow, practical, and inspirational guide that provides a background to the nature and range of dreams and reveals the power of dream interpretation.

$14.95 • Paper • ISBN 0-89594-966-0

Essential Reiki: A Complete Guide to an Ancient Healing Art
By Diane Stein

This bestseller includes the history of Reiki, hand positions, giving treatments, and the initiations. While no book can replace directly received attunements, Essential Reiki provides everything else that the practitioner and teacher of this system needs, including all three degrees of Reiki, most of it in print for the first time.

$18.95 • Paper • ISBN 0-89594-736-6

BOOKS BY THE CROSSING PRESS

Essential Reiki: A Complete Guide to an Ancient Healing Art

By Diane Stein

This bestseller includes the history of Reiki, hand positions, giving treatments, and the initiations. While no book can replace directly received attunements, Essential Reiki provides everything else that the practitioner and teacher of this system needs, including all three degrees of Reiki, most of it in print for the first time.

$18.95 • Paper • ISBN 0-89594-736-6

Fundamentals of Hawaiian Mysticism

By Charlotte Berney

Evolving in isolation on an island paradise, the mystical practice of Huna has shaped the profound yet elegantly simple Hawaiian character. Charlotte Berney presents Huna traditions as they apply to words, prayer, gods, the breath, a loving spirit, family ties, nature, and mana.

$12.95 • Paper • ISBN 1-58091-026-2

Fundamentals of Jewish Mysticm and Kabbalah

By Ron Feldman

This concise introductory book explains what Kabbalah is and how study of its text and practices enhance the life of the soul and the holiness of the body.

$12.95 • Paper • ISBN 1-58091-049-1

Fundamentals of Tibetan Buddhism

By Rebecca McClen Novick

This book explores the history, philosophy, and practice of Tibetan Buddhism. Novick's concise history of Buddhism, and her explanations of the Four Noble Truths, Wheel of Life, Karma, Five Paths, Six Perfections, and the different schools of thought within the Buddhist teachings help us understand Tibetan Buddhism as a way of experiencing the world, more than as a religion or philosophy.

$12.95 • Paper • ISBN 0-89594-953-9

The Healing Energy of Your Hands

By Michael Bradford

Bradford offers techniques so simple that anyone can work with healing energy quickly and easily.

$12.95 • Paper • ISBN 0-89594-781-1

Gandhi's Health Guide

By Mahatma Gandhi

Many people may not know that Gandhi's thoughts on health are as original as his thoughts on spirituality and politics. His inquiring mind led him to dispense with the pills he used daily and discover what truly benefited his family's health. Discover how Gandhi's renunciation of Western medicine transformed the man and his ideas.

$12.95 • Paper • ISBN 1-58091-051-3

BOOKS BY THE CROSSING PRESS

The Language of Dreams

By Patricia Telesco

Patricia Telesco outlines a creative, interactive approach to understanding the dream symbols of our inner life. Interpretations of more than 800 dream symbols incorporate multi-cultural elements with psychological, religious, folk, and historical meanings.

$16.95 • Paper • ISBN 0-89594-836-2

Old Age Is Another Country: A Traveler's Guide

By Page Smith

A bit of clear thinking on some age-old questions about old age.—Kirkus Reviews

$12.95 • Paper • ISBN 0-89594-776-5

Pocket Guide to Chakras

By Joy Gardner-Gordon

This book will answer your questions about chakra, including explaining what they are, where they are, how they function and what causes the chakras to open and close.

$6.95 • Paper • ISBN 0-89594-949-0

Pocket Guide to Hatha Yoga

By Michele Picozzi

Hatha yoga is a holistic form of exercise tailor-made for modern Westerners. This guide offers a roadmap for the beginner and a comprehensive resource for the continuing yoga student.

$6.95 • Paper • ISBN 0-89594-911-3

Pocket Guide to Meditation

By Alan Pritz

This book focuses on meditation as part of spiritual practice, as a universal tool to forge a deeper connection with spirit. In Alan Pritz's words, Meditation simply delivers one of the most purely profound experiences of life, joy.

$6.95 • Paper • ISBN 0-89594-886-9

Pocket Guide to Stress Reduction

By Brenda O'Hanlon

This take-along guide provides a useful checklist to assess your stress level and teaches you various ways to reduce your stress. Learn how to manage, harness, and control the stress in your life rather than allowing it to control you.

$6.95 • Paper • ISBN 1-58091-011-4

BOOKS BY THE CROSSING PRESS

Pocket Guide to Visualization
By Helen Graham

Visualization is imagining; producing mental images that come to mind as pictures we can see. These pictures can help you relax, assess and manage stress, improve self-awareness, alleviate disease and manage pain.

$6.95 • Paper • ISBN 0-89594-885-0

Recurring Dreams: A Journey to Wholeness
By Kathleen Sullivan

Are you troubled by a dream that repeats its message again and again, sometimes over a period of years? What is the dream trying to tell you? Kathleen Sullivan shows you ways to transform your life through exploring your dreams.

$16.95 • Paper • ISBN 0-89594-892-3

Resolving Conflict Sooner: The Powerfully Simple 4-Step Method for Reaching Better Agreements More Easily in Everyday Life
By Kare Anderson

Kare Anderson gives us 4 simple steps to *Resolving Conflict Sooner.* Through these four simple steps, Kare shows us how conflict can be an opportunity for people to come together, connect, and establish a deeper connection.

$10.95 • Paper • ISBN 0-89594-976-8

Writing from the Heart: Inspiration and Exercises for Women Who Want to Write
By Leslea Newman

There's more to this book than inspiration. For presenting the basics of writing structure and technique, this book has few peers.—Lambda Book Report

$14.95 • Paper • ISBN 0-89594-641-6

Your Body Speaks Your Mind: How Your thoughts and Emotions Affect Your Health
By Debbie Shapiro

Debbie Shapiro examines the intimate connection between the mind and body revealing insights into how our unresolved thoughts and feelings affect our health and manifest as illness in specific parts of the body.

$14.95 • Paper • ISBN 0-89594-893-1

To receive a current catalog from The Crossing Press
please call toll-free, 800-777-1048.
Visit our Web site: **www.crossingpress.com**